The Neuropsychology of Developmental Stuttering

In memory of:
Alfred Abrahamsen
Jens Abrahamsen
Sam Block Sandved

The Neuropsychology of Developmental Stuttering

A Psychosocial Approach to Understanding and Treating Developmental Stuttering

Bernard-thomas Hartman, PhD
ASLHA: CCC: Speech pathology

W
Whurr Publishers Ltd
London

First published 1994 by
Whurr Publishers Ltd
19B Compton Terrace, London N1 2UN, England

British Library Cataloguing-in-Publication Data
A catalogue record for this book is available from the British Library

ISBN 1-897635-46-X

Photoset by Stephen Cary
Printed and bound in the UK by Athenæum Press Ltd., Gateshead, Tyne & Wear.

Preface

During my earlier years as a speech pathologist, I achieved moderately sucessful therapy results, particularly with stutterers who were either in their late teens or adults. Although often exhibiting increased fluent speech within the clinical setting, clients still reported consistent difficulties in their daily experiences, in spite of self-administration of techniques learned in the clinic. It was becoming apparent that therapy methods for mainly treating their stuttering behaviors had definite remedial limitations. These difficulties were confirmed in discussions with other therapists.

The search for the means to obtain better results led me to review how young children develop speech. My attention was drawn to certain basic factors:

- Speech-gratification experiences derived from the successes of their speech efforts motivated and reinforced their dependence on speech.
- Children normally developed speech with little need to be consciously preoccupied or concerned with either its on-going development or the manner of their speech performance.
- The basic functions of speech develop as automated neurophysiological motor processes.

Over 2000 years ago, Demosthenes, a stutterer and noted Athenian statesman and orator, used the distraction of pebbles, complemented with the masking background of the roaring surf against the seashore, as a means to effect fluent speech. He noted that he did not stutter when speaking against a noisy background because he could not hear himself speak. (He had no need to, because speech functions develop as *automated* neurophysiological motor processes.) Consequently, he experienced *speech gratifications* from the success of his efforts. Also his concern for swallowing the pebbles while speaking distracted him from *'undo' preoccupations* with his speech.

Since Demosthenes, stutterers have been subjected to an awesome assortment of methods employed to cure, control, suppress, repress, exorcise, etc. the disruptive effects of their stuttering behaviors on the fluency of their developed speech. Most of these methods provided no beneficial results, although some obtained mild to moderate, although often inconsistent, results.

Among the surviving methods currently employed are distraction and masking techniques – some closely akin to those used by Demosthenes. Considering our advanced knowledge of stuttering, and our sophisticated means for implementation of these techniques, it would seem that, whether by design or not, certain factors contributing to Demosthenes' successful self-therapy are not accounted for within most clinical programs.

Current clinical programs generally adhere to long-held therapy methods that stutterers must self-administer to control, circumvent, desensitize, unlearn, etc. their disturbed fluency behaviors. These methods therefore mainly treat these behaviors, rather than the *conditions* that foster their repeated occurrences. These methods seem intent on separating the stutterer from his or her dysfluency behaviors.

Furthermore, these methods require the client's constant attention, if they are to be properly self-administered, particularly outside the clinical setting. This can inadvertently lead to the 'undo' preoccupations particularly concerning: self-administration of the required techniques; the effectiveness of the techniques on speech performance; and anticipation relative to the outcome of speech efforts to obtain *gratification of desired objectives*.

These preoccupations are seen to be contrary to the normal automated functions of the individual's developed neurophysiological motor processes for producing speech. They may contribute not only to the severity of the stuttering behaviors, but also to the conditions that promote their repeated occurrences.

Stuttering is not a developmental or organic disorder of speech, as is evident in the stutterer's ability to produce fluent speech. Stuttering cannot therefore be treated by the mechanistic/manipulation methods more common to treatment of disorders of speech. It is a psychosocial behavioral disorder, manifesting periodic non-speech motor behaviors triggered by disturbed perceptions of, and traumatic neuropsychological reactions to, particular external conditions within certain situations; these disrupt the forward flow of developed fluent speech.

If clinical programs are to obtain more consistent beneficial results from therapy, they should endeavor, as this book recommends, to treat more directly the negative psychosocial conditions that sustain and promote loss of ready availability of the stutterer's developed fluent speech.

Bernard-thomas Hartmann
July 1994

Contents

Acknowledgments

This book represents the product of valuable assistance and resources contributed by many people, and entrusted to the author to organize and present in a respectable and enlightened form. It is hoped that this book does credit to their trust, and serves all those for whom it has been written.

Special thanks go to Rolf Gerhardt, former Chief of the Psychological Services, Royal Norwegian Armed Forces, for insights into possible comparative neurophysiological connections between dyslexia and stuttering and for his suggestions based on extensive experience with dyslexia and related perceptual–motor disorders.

I would also like to show my appreciation to Jan Stolp, Health and Sosialsjef, Oppland Fylkeskommune, Lillehammer, Norway; The Lillehammer Fylkessykehus; and Per Slaastuen, Sjef-psykolog, Psykiaktrisk Klinikken, for providing opportunities to pursue this study.

In addition appreciation is extended to the following:

Reidar Eriksen, Rektor, Halmrast Senter for Stamme-behandling; Else Halmrast, Kontorsjef; Tom Green, Spesialpsykolog; Marie Øfstaas, Boligsjef, Kåra Ofstaas, former Rector, and other staff members for their gracious and consistent support.

Special gratitude to the residents, young and old, attending the Halmrast Senter, who offered friendship, trust and cooperation.

To Asle Hovdahl, Rektor; Ulv Lassen, Rektor; Torstein Lundbekk, Kontorsjef, and to Janne Johansson, Avdelingsleder, Engehagen, Senter for Utviklingshemmede, Gjøvik, for resources and encouragement.

To Gardner Gately, Chairman, Department of Communication Sciences, Baylor University, and Tom Brennan, Speech and Hearing Pathologist, Nacogdoches, Texas, for the many mind-bending discussions, progressive ideas and uncommon commonsense.

To Annette Orynauka, and the many students, who during many pleasant years with the Speech and Hearing Clinic, Stephen F. Austin

State University, Texas, privileged me by using me as their mentor, and for learning from them.

To the many clients for their consistent trust in our programs.
To many colleagues: Thad Paruzynski, Department of Communication Disorders, Marquette University, Wisconsin; Dr Richard Voigtel, Chairman, Counseling and Special Educational Programs, Stephen F. Austin State University, Texas; Roger Sandeklev, Sjefpsykolog, Barne-og Ungdomspsykiatrisk Poliklinikk, Oppland Fylkeskommune, Gjøvik, Norway.

Above all, to my wife, Berit, and sons – Edward, John and Brian – for their invaluable encouragement, patience and assistance, which made the inevitable difficulties manageable; the many long hours of research and writing companionable; and a most capricious computer functional; and tante Randi Sandved; I affectionately dedicate this book to them, with love.

Chapter 1
Setting the stage

Introduction

'Hear me now and believe me later' is an expression popularized on the American comedy TV show 'Saturday Nite Live'. The seeming absurdity of this expression may well hide the wisdom of its subtle plea, which could speak for those of us who believe we have something worth saying, if only we could be heard.

This book is such a desire to be heard, if what it relates is to be believed. There may be nothing unique about a speech pathologist, a psychologist, an audiologist, a special educator or even a stutterer writing a book on stuttering. Still, maybe one of us has learned a thing or two about stuttering worth listening to – if what is said is to be believed.

This book was not written just for stutterers, who probably know more about their problems, if only others had the patience to listen to them. It was also written for: students and practitioners of speech pathology, psychologists, medical and related professional disciplines, educators, politicians, and, above all, anybody inclined to listen with patience and interest. Stuttering, also referred to as stammering, has a unique, strange, sometimes weird and all too often unpleasant history. The term 'developmental stuttering' is generally credited to Brutten (1969). For the purpose of brevity, stuttering is used when developmental stuttering is referred to.

Few behavioral disorders have presented such a puzzling challenge to so many different professional disciplines. Stuttering still continues to be regarded, however, as an enigma wrapped within a mystery with respect to its etiological, psychosocial and remedial bases. Stuttering has been subjected to extensive and intensive research during the last 70 years, with accumulation of many data. Much has been learned about this confounding human behavioral disorder, and yet it remains subject to considerable speculation, controversy, misunderstanding and misrepresentation.

Stuttering continues to be treated as a most complex and puzzling form of disturbed human behavior. Years of training, research and treating stutterers have, however, led me to view stuttering as somewhat less complex and puzzling, and to draw conclusions supported by these experiences. These conclusions relate, in large part, to certain aspects of the neurophysiology and neuropsychology of stuttering that may not be generally known or that are considered to be of minimal, if any, importance to the understanding or treatment of stuttering, particularly with respect to teenage and adult stutterers.

In the following chapters, attention is paid to certain neurophysiological and neuropsychological factors that are deemed to be intimately associated with the formation and repeated episodes of stuttering behaviors. These factors will be shown to support the notion that stuttering behaviors do not inhibit the development of the neurophysiological motor processes for speech production; in addition, they do not alter developed motor speech processes. Rather, stuttering behaviors are regarded as disruptive episodes to the ready availability and forward synchronous flow of the individual's developed fluent speech performances. This notion, and the contention, that stuttering, as a psychosocial behavioral disorder, is a neuropsychological phenomenon are central to the objectives of this book, which proposes insights towards advancing the understanding and treatment of teenage and adult stutterers.

Even if the cause(s) for stuttering could be determined definitively, it is doubtful that total prevention of stuttering could be realized. We might, therefore, deal with the reality that today there are millions who stutter, and that the future probability is of millions of others. These millions represent human beings with resources of intelligence and talent, who are no different from non-stutterers. This intelligence and talent will continue to be compromised through public ignorance and/or misunderstanding, and the limitations that clinical programs have in providing beneficial and consistent therapy results.

Notations

The reader will note repetition of certain topics; this is to enable the readers to be aware of the roles and influences of these topics on the major themes of this book. It is hoped the readers will also find these helpful, rather than unduly distracting.

The reader may also note that references to children and adults are commonly in the male gender. No chauvinism is intended, because women can also be afflicted with stuttering behaviors and subjected to the same consequences. Unfortunately, over the last five decades or so, the incidence of stuttering among women is regarded to have risen significantly towards the higher level generally assessed for males.

Extensive research has been undertaken in writing this book, but it has been difficult to provide references to support all statements and conclusions. Who can remember all the sources for what he has *learned* or *reasoned* from training and related experiences? Although large numbers of references are provided, it is deemed unproductive and unduly distracting to flood each page with references. This does not indicate a lack of respect or appreciation for those authors who have commented on the topics; I am indebted to them for whatever successes this book may realize in its move towards a better understanding and treatment of stutterers.

Furthermore, certain topics, ideas, statements and conclusions might appear to be somewhat simplistic, overly contentious or, possibly, outright fantastic. It is hoped, however, that readers will view the contents of this book with an open mind; as someone much wiser wrote:

> When a closed mind is re-opened, it may still be under the same management.

Background commentaries on stuttering:

> Stuttering, as a speech defect, arrests the attention of all who come into casual contact with it, and enlists the interest of all associated with the stutterer:
> It challenges the speech pathologist's spirit of research.
> It tasks the ingenuity of the scrupulous, conscientious clinician.
> It furnishes a harvest for the charlatan.
> It appeals to the sentimental.
> Above all, it hampers the – stutterer.
>
> *West, Kennedy and Carr (1937)*

The above comments on the general attitudes towards stuttering were written nearly 60 years ago. Such comments could well have been written today to express current attitudes towards stuttering and stutterers, in spite of the great increase in university, college, public school and private clinic programs for treating stuttering behaviors. There has also been extensive research on stuttering. Although much of this research has been competent, there has also been an apparently strong compulsive and mundane search for all manner of etiological, as well as pathological and functional, deficits to account for, or attribute to, stutterering. In spite of their apparent absurdity, the persistent pursuit of such questionable research often produced strange contradictions and misconceptions; this brings to mind an anecdote illustrating the general slant of such research.

> A man was observed searching intently under a street light. Another man walking by stopped and inquired, 'Did you lose something? Perhaps I can help?'

'Yes, perhaps you can. I lost my car keys somewhere over there,' the man answered, pointing to a dark area some distance from the street light.

'But, why then,' asked the startled pedestrian, 'do you search for them over here?'

'Obviously,' the man answered, showing impatience, 'because the light is better here.'

The stutterer: to be or not to be handicapped?

During the 1960s and 1970s, civil rights movements, with legal encouragement, have stirred the public to accept long overdue responsibilities towards its handicapped members. Although these movements fostered benefits for many handicapped people, attention to the needs of adult stutterers was overlooked. Quite possibly, the legislators, and professional disciplines, had difficulty clearly defining what constitutes a handicap and what being disadvantaged means. This distinction, whether imposed directly or indirectly, is all too often a fact of life for many stutterers, particularly adults; these adults are disadvantaged from their potentials to succeed and as a result are caused to be handicapped. What is written below about general attitudes towards and treatment of stutterers could well apply to other groups.

Webster's New World Dictionary (1968) defines *handicap* as:

Something that *hampers* a person; a disdvantage; a hindrance.
To *cause* to be at a *disadvantage*; to hinder; to impede.

On consideration of the above definitions, we may see a significant difference between *being hampered by a handicap*, and *being caused to be handicapped through being disadvantaged*. A person might be blind, deaf, epileptic, palsied or different in color, race or religion, etc. Or, he might stutter. Although society does not always determine rightly what constitutes a handicap, it does, however, generally determine who is disadvantaged and thus set apart from society's mainstream.

Modern societies tend to regard stuttering with a certain *ambivalence*. When children attending school exhibit stuttering behaviors, there is generally some cause for concern and public therapy programs, when available, are often provided. Adult stutterers, however, often tend to be *disadvantaged*, not only from opportunities to pursue personal, social and vocational aspirations, but from public therapy assistance. This might possibly reflect an unintentional bias to which Dr Seuss might have commented:

Adult stutterers are simply children who have gone bad.

People are generally well-meaning and could well be surprised and/or discomforted to be made aware of the extent to which they have inadvertently contributed to the formation and sustainment of an individual's stuttering behaviors. Also, through misguided attitudes and related acts, they could have contributed to stutterers being disadvantaged from personal, social and/or vocational opportunities that they commonly expect to be accorded to themselves.

The general public usually relies on its professional members for information relating to health, education and welfare. Professionals can greatly influence public attitudes towards those members exhibiting various forms of physical, mental or behavioral disorders, particularly when such disorders are purported to be based on research. When professionals, through assessment, have foisted on stutterers an almost endless list of inherent pathologies, functional symptoms and deficits, what impressions should the public form about stutterers? The absurdity of many of these assessments has become so apparent that Bloodstein (1975), a leading authority on stuttering, has expressed his concerns as follows:

> Can the 'typical stutterer' be depicted to be: anally fixated, brain-damaged with atypical cortical dominance, inadequate of sound-mindedness; to possess inter-aural-phase disparities, lower auditory pain thresholds, vascular and biochemical imbalances, and/or a multiple of other differential anomalies?

An attitude often put upon stutterers is one of ***benevolent avoidance***. This attitude reflects a general tendency on the part of the public to avoid making direct commitments to the stutterer; this is often true regarding the stutterer's needs and aspirations which, in view of ***misperceived speech limitations*** and other deficits, are deemed to be impractical and not in his best interests. Stutterers, particularly older teenagers and adults, are often beset with this perplexing and frustrating dilemma. They are often advised to be realistic, and to accept and live with what is generally ***unacceptable*** to others, namely their stuttering behaviors. Such counseling tends to reflect a kind of general ***public hubris***.

Comments: the general public and professionals should therefore understand the extent to which misguided attitudes and actions contribute, directly or indirectly, towards disadvantaging those members who have stuttering behaviors. There are many who stuttered and yet contributed to the arts, sciences, education, industry and other fields. It is grossly erroneous to contend that they succeeded in spite of their stuttering. On the contrary, they succeeded because they had the intelligence and talent to do so. As for non-stutterers, they were permitted or able to make the opportunities succeed. Their contributions should confirm the loss of potential talent of those numbers of stutterers who are disadvantaged.

Stutterers, in persistent search of cure

Stutterers are generally ever hopeful of an end to their stuttering behaviors, and the restrictions such behaviors impose on them. Adult stutterers, in particular those who have failed to gain beneficial therapy results from prior participation in clinic programs, tend to be susceptible to *pseudo-professional* programs promising them freedom from the bondage of their imprisoned speech. They are therefore prone to enter such programs at costs they can ill-afford or to try again – just one more time – in spite of the limited beneficial or consistent results experienced in similar programs.

There are often *pseudo-religious connotations* to these programs. One nationally syndicated program that promised to cure stuttering offers two-day workshops usually held at a local motel. Current costs are about US$2300, plus travelling and living expenses. Post-workshop counselling, paradoxically, is provided by telephone, for a limited period. Administration of this program is restricted only to its guru and his disciples, who have been ordained into the guru's training program, usually at a cost of about US$1800, plus cumulative expenses. The techniques applied are regarded as secretive. Yet, they tend to be similar to methods used in past and current clinic programs, some of which are deemed inadequate. The failure of clients to benefit from the program is regarded as the result of *lack of complete spiritual faith in the guru and program*. There are no refunds.

There are similar quasi-professional programs promoting *mail-order, home, self-therapy programs*, which use various forms of TV and other assortments of book-cassettes or devices. In spite of sanctions imposed by the Ethics Committee of the American Speech–Language and Hearing Association, and restrictions of state legislation, such workshops continue to prosper through legal loopholes.

Stuttering: puzzling resistance to remedial approaches

The search for means to cure or control stuttering behaviors has challenged the ingenuity of many professional disciplines for a long time. This elusive search has led to a mind-bending array of professional and quasi-professional remedial approaches, ranging from witchcraft and exorcism to current manipulative methods, and masking feedback devices. In spite of this extensive diversification of remedial approaches, stuttering continues to be resistant to varying degrees to therapy techniques.

Some of the more dominant of past and current approaches are:

- Restrictive oral devices for limiting tongue and jaw movements: often painful.
- Oral surgery: clipping of the tongue and/or lingua frenum.
- Exorcism and related faith healing rites.
- Hypnotism (including postsuggestive states).
- Neurosurgery.
- Nutrition.
- Drugs.
- Chiropractics.
- Oral-manipulation drills.
- Autosuggestive techniques.
- Sociodrama.
- Desensitization methods.
- Rote drill methods.
- Classical conditioning methods.
- Behavior modification (operant techniques).
- Biofeedback methods.
- Delayed auditory feedback.
- Relaxation and related bodily control methods.
- Acupuncture.
- Transcendental meditation and related techniques.
- Avoidance and/or distraction techniques.
- Psychotherapy/psychoanalysis approaches.
- Mental visualization methods.
- Assorted psychological approaches.
- Guidance/counselling methods.
- Self-help therapy methods.
- Auditory masking devices.
- Voice-masking devices.
- Neuropsychology approach.

Although some of the above remedial approaches have proved to be more beneficial with other forms of behavioral disorders, relatively few have gained any modicum of success with stutterers. Many others were found to be ineffective, and still others to be painful and quite harmful, for example, the use of oral devices, which used sharp spikes to control the speaker's tongue movements. Most certainly, witch hunts or the use of surgical methods brought little joy or relief.

Martin and Seigal (1966), using antecedent stimulus control with operant conditioning techniques, reported that, using illumination from a blue light, the subjects showed reduced stuttering behaviors. The value of such studies, which attempt to determine reduced stuttering behaviors by methods failing to consider adaptation affects, within controlled and meaningless environments, tends to be subject to considerable doubt.

The neuropsychology of human behavior

Seemingly, new ideas may not be new, but are in fact old ideas that have lain dormant. The basic concepts concerning the neuropsychology of human behavior have been floating about the humanistic classrooms and laboratories within universities and colleges for the last 60 years. Only during recent years has significant attention been directed towards neuropsychology as a potentially advantageous approach to the treatment, as well as the study, of certain types of behavioral disorders. More recently, interest has been shown in the application of neuropsychology to stuttering.

The concepts of neuropsychology are founded on the premise that *external influences can influence the organization and functions of neurons within the brain, thus affecting the performances of* specific skills and behaviors. The brain continues its structural development, particularly with regard to its complexes of associated neural networks, during the years after an infant's birth. This development after birth depends greatly on external stimuli. Consequently, *external stimuli can influence the child's behavioral developments significantly during his early formative years*. External stimuli have also been shown to influence brain functions and therefore the child's behavior throughout his life.

Neuropsychology traces its formal beginnings to the works of a father and son – R.A. Luria and A.R. Luria – in Russia before the Second World War. At that time, the Lurias worked under the very severe regimentation imposed by the communist state on its scientific community. The Soviets placed great emphasis on research into human behaviors, which they subordinated to the rigid dictates of the prevailing Marxist–Leninist doctrines, which maintained that the state, through design of its external regimen, could alter *genetic specificity*, so shaping and controlling human behavior (Cole, 1978).

Before the Second World War, it was generally accepted that the *right side* of the brain was subject mainly to control by the *dominant left side*. The Lurias concluded, from their studies of *aphasic behaviors*, that this was not only an error, but that the right hemisphere controlled the crucial powers of recognizing reality, which every creature must have in order to survive (Cole, 1978).

The Lurias contended that an essential aspect of these crucial powers of recognizing reality related directly to the ability to *perceive cognitively* and *mediate performance according to the person's environmental experiences*. Goldstein (1948) regarded this, as did the Lurias, to be a primary problem for aphasic individuals resulting from brain injury. Failure to do so might well constitute a threat to the *person's well-being, if not to outright survival*.

These concepts questioned the strong attention being paid to the left hemisphere, as the dominant control center for learning (Rosenthal, 1977). As expected, there was considerable opposition to this ascendancy of the right hemisphere as an important center for learning.

These findings were based on studies of relatively unknown functions of neural areas within the right hemisphere, which were found to be extremely sensitive to the individual's cognitive perceptions and responses, subject to his environmental experiences.

These concepts seemingly competed with the long-held emphasis on genetics as the dominant determinator of higher human skills and behaviors. The communists contended that these concepts confirmed the dialectics of their doctrines, which claimed that genetically based characteristics, used in the formation of skills and behaviors, could be altered and regulated by regimentation of external environments. The Lurias, however, never believed that external stimuli could so completely dominate, let alone negate, human genetic specificity. In later papers, they acknowledged the *relative rigidity* of genetics (Luria, 1966a).

The Lurias, however, did not disavow their neuropsychological concepts, which considered the effective influences of external stimuli on learning. On the contrary, they asserted that children were indeed very dependent on external influences for the formative outcome of their genetically specified skills and behaviors. Learning, the Lurias contended, requires continuous and harmonious interplay between the genetically specified neurons for the particular skills, and the children's on-going perceptions of external experiences.

In summary, the pursuit of studies in neuropsychology may well provide an innovative means of shedding light on unknown aspects of our limited understanding of behavior disorders, such as stuttering, and its cumulative psychosocial affects on people so afflicted. The general public would be quite surprised at how well stutterers would appear with a little light directed towards their darkened corners.

Rolf Gerhardt: perceptual–motor concepts

All knowledge to be learned, first must be perceived by the senses.

Aristotle

Rolf Gerhardt, former Chief of Psychological Services of the Royal Norwegian Armed Forces, has studied extensively the effects of perceptual–motor disorders on pilots, and on adults and children with reading disabilities. From these studies, Gerhardt (1977) contended that there might be a *possible etiological relationship* between *dyslexia* (a reading disorder) and *stuttering*, because both disorders involve basic communication skills and require proper perceptions, and temporal sequencing of neurophysiological processes for their many perceptual–motor movements.

I do not intend to attempt either to *support* or to *negate* the possibility of an *etiological* connection between dyslexia and stuttering. However, I do wonder whether or not the drawing of primitive pictures by the earliest humans might have preceded speech through the attachment of primordial vocalizations to the pictures. Gerhardt did, however, acknowledge that considerably more research is required before a definite conclusion can be reached.

There may, however, be a valid connection between dyslexia and stuttering, when considering the *comparative similarities* in the formation of disturbed *neurophysiological motor processes* and the temporal sequencing of their perceptual–motor movements. Gerhardt contended that there were comparative similarities in the formation of the neurophysiological perceptual–motor processes with regard to performances of both *normal and disturbed reading skills*. Furthermore, he regarded *external influences* as dominant in the formation of both normal reading and dyslexic disorders, and assumed a similar relationship between normal speech and stuttering.

Gerhardt maintained, in addition, that changes in the organization and function of specific neural cell assemblies are usually the result of characteristic patterns of sensorineural excitations generated by the perceptual sensory–modality (perceptual–motor) systems. Clear and consistent perceptions will be reflected in the normal formation and performances of the particular skill. If the perceptions are ambiguous, the performances of the skill will also tend to appear ambiguous. Based on his extensive work with dyslexia and related perceptual–motor disorders, Gerhardt (1977) concluded:

> Variations in the formation of the 'directional laterality' of perceptual–motor movements (processes), might alone account for the significant differences found in children and adults, deemed to be 'free of inherent or acquired defects'.

Gerhardt, and Fitts, regarded the formation of genetically specific skills to consist of the following components: neurogenic, neurophysiologcal and neuropsychological.

The neurogenic components

These comprise the organizations of neural cell assemblies, which possess the genetic specificity for skills and behaviors, within the various cortical levels of the brain.

The neurophysiological components

These comprise the perceptual–motor system, with its perception modalities: assemblies of neurons and their motor cells, the neural synaptic connectors and associative nerve fibers, and the muscular and skeletal systems. These components implement the temporal sequences of perceptual–motor movement patterns relative to the neurophysiological performances of specific skills or behaviors.

The neuropsychological components

These consist of the cognitive systems within the higher cortical levels of the brain. These systems relate to the recognition of reality, intellect, sensation and emotional systems. These systems are particularly sensitive to *external stimuli* and can therefore affect the organization and function of the neurophysiological components.

Gerhardt (1977) regarded breakdowns in the interplay between the above components and external stimuli as disruptive to the temporal sequencing of the perceptual–motor patterns formed within the neurophysiological components. He considered this to be evident in the disturbed writing performances of young schoolchildren, whose disturbed perceptual–motor processes negatively affected the organization of neurons and their motor cells, which genetically specify the basic performances of writing skill. (For more detailed information about Gerhardt, see Appendix I.)

> *Comments*: it is contended that the selective influence of external stimuli on the neurophysiological formation of specific basic skills, such as reading, can also be related to motor speech performances, such as fluent speech. It is contended further that stuttering behaviors, which can be likened to reading disorders, can also be subject to comparatively similar neurophysiological formations in individuals who are 'free of prior inherent or acquired defects'; this might account for their occurrence. These two basic assumptions are closely relevant to the major themes of this book

Human genetic specificity for speech, reading and other basic skills

> We are committed to speak, because we are human.
>
> *Rose (1973)*

There is general agreement that humans and many other lower life forms possess the genetic specificity for speech or other forms of communication. Studies have determined that many lower life forms share with humans distinctively elaborate speech–sound systems than was once believed (*Newsweek*, 23 May 1988).

These studies report that the speech–sound systems possessed by these lower life forms are not merely instinctive vocal reflexes of arousal or warning, but fairly detailed reports of events of their world. News commentators apparently also mutate among lower life forms. What could they be reporting about human events?

Theological teachings have long regarded humans as being singularly predominant in their inherent specificity for higher skills. Research studies, however, which assert the genetic specificity of the human brain for developing higher basic skills, such as speech, reading, writing, etc., are of relatively recent vintage. The Lurias held that the processes by which children learn to read and write do not begin within their classrooms, but rather are contingent upon two primary factors:

1. The pre-history of the biological evolution towards the development of these higher forms of human skills.
2. The earliest attainment and assimilation of skills and abilities which will have enabled the children to master reading and writing skills within the relatively short period of time they are expected to do so.

Cole (1978)

Hebb (1956) maintained that humans, within their conceptual systems, have the genetic potential to develop perceptual skills. He correlated the activities of individual neurons (nerve cells) with identifiable neurophysiological phenomena, and offered the following comment:

> The primitive perceptual unity and segregation from the background appears to be a native capacity of sensory excitations, and the inherited characteristics of the nervous system.

Chomsky (1957, cited in Rose, 1973) considered language acquisition to be innovatively specific. He does, however, appear to place less genetic importance on the developmental sequences related to children's acquisition of language, or with regard to the interactions of such developmental sequences with their environments. Although genetic specificity for language is regarded as an inherent potential, it is nevertheless, as the Lurias stated, subject to environmental influences for the manner of its development. Although in agreement with this, Chomsky contended that language also appears to be a common denominator among many forms of mammals, as well as in humans, each, however, having different levels of 'genetically-wired neural systems for language acquisition' (Rose, 1973).

Piaget's concept of genetic epistemology, however, proposed that children's skills were 'wired-in genetically in sequences of their development from the neural tube to the cerebral cortex'. Piaget further maintained that the infant's sequences of behavioral events, beginning with its first smile, and ending with logical and abstract concepts, were also wired-in genetically. The infant thus, in the development of his ability to process and analyze language, and in his approach to the world behaviorally, was genetically wired (Rose, 1973).

Rose, however, disagreed with Piaget's genetically wired-in notion of the infant's developmental sequences of behavioral events. He stated that this appeared to overly robotize the infant's sequential formation of behavioral events. If infants are so genetically wired-in, then why are their behavioral events so differentially responsive to environmental stimuli? Rose applied genetic epistemology to human development in its more classical context. He regarded genetic epistemology as:

> The study of the way bodies of knowledge grow and become organized to the extent knowledge, observations, and analytical techniques, placed at the disposal of the individual possessing the genetic-potentials, are being developed.

The difference between these two approaches is more than merely semantics. Whereas Piaget regarded human functions, such as language and consciousness, to be so genetically wired that they are properties of the brain, Rose regarded them as properties of the organism possessing the brain. In reference to this Rose stated:

> It would be foolish for the brain to possess genetic potentials for higher functions, without the organism's having the neural networks, and related motor systems, to permit their development and usage.

Rose further maintained that, even if higher skills might be wired-in as genetically specific, they nevertheless should be considered as potentials that are subject to the individual's experiences after birth and, thus, effectively influenced by environmental conditions. Rose's statements about the infant's genetic specificity for higher skills are considered more consistent with the basic concepts of neuropsychology. Higher skills, such as speech, reading, etc., do not appear to be 'wired-in as pre-programmed tapes', to be activated at various stages of the infant's development.

Gerhardt, in further support of this, maintained that genetic specificity for higher skills was evident in the rigidity of the neural assemblies for retaining and exhibiting the basic formations of the particular skill, in spite of severe levels of functional disturbance to the skill. In this regard he stated:

> Disruptive influences tend to selectively affect the formation of specific skills, rather than constitute a generalized disturbance to the formation of a variety of other skills.

Hebb (1950) expressed the relationships between neurogenic components and learning, as follows:

> Learning is the product of intricate, yet highly dependent relationships established between the child's 'genetic-specificity' for basic human skills, and the complex interneuronal associations of the brain levels. It is within these relationships that the nervous system fulfils its potentials to selectively identify and respond to a seemingly unlimited range of internal and external simuli.

In summary, humans inherently possess the genetic specificities for basic skills. Speech is regarded as one of the more dominant of these skills. Humans depend upon speech as the primary communicative medium for forming, binding and perpetuating their societal systems. Speech can, however, functionally influence, as well as be subject to, socioenvironmental stimuli.

Genetic specificity and environmental influences

The Lurias (Luria, 1966a,b) contended, as noted earlier, that the interactions between genetic specificity and environmental stimuli are the basis for the neuropsychological approach to the formation of human skills and behaviors. Although humans possess a most remarkable range of genetically specified skills and behaviors, their dependence on external stimuli is evident in their wonderful productions in art, literature, music, medicine, as well as ingenious means of industrialization, agriculture, communications, travel, etc. Humans, unlike other life forms, however, also possess the inherent potentials to apply their remarkable skills just as ingeniously to self-destruction.

Humans, as social organisms, generally strive to provide themselves with a secure, stable, communal environment. Human societies, however, are prone to grow and change, which increases and alters the nature of the environmental influences greatly affecting the lives of its members, and the directional development and use of their remarkable genetic potentials.

Learning basic perceptual–motor skills, such as reading and speech, thus requires attending to the interactive relationships between the perceptual–motor movements fostered by perceptions of the external stimuli, and their functional effects upon the motoneurons for the specific skill (Gerhardt, 1977).

Comments: the effects of environmental influence on the members of a society are particularly germane to the neuropsychology of human learning and behavior. This relates to the behavioral psychosocial consequences that environmental influences can impose on individual members, groups of members or society as a whole.

The plasticity of the human nervous system

This refers to the ability of assemblies of neurons and their synaptic connectors to change their levels of resistance to sensory excitations. When repeatedly activated, these assemblies of neurons become preferentially sensitized (less resistant) to activation by particular sensory excitations.

All life forms contain genes and chromosome – the genetic blueprints which, as rigid genetic determinators for replication, assure hereditary reproduction of the particular biological lineage of the species. These blueprints, depending on the nature of the species, can relate to either singular or a combination of genetically specific determinators for basic behavior and/or skills.

These behaviors and/or skills exhibited by many lower life forms, although quite remarkable, are nevertheless unlearned. Rather they are products of rigid genetic specificity, more commonly referred to as instincts

Still, we marvel at the remarkable geometric consistency of the inner structures of the beehive; the tensile, yet delicate lacework of the spider's web; or the intricate maze of tunnels and well-defined social order of the ant colony. Each generation of these lower species performs its particular skills without any apparent post-birth learning. In addition to replicating their basic inherent genetic characteristics, higher life forms, and humans in particular, also possess genetically specified potentials for higher forms of skills and behaviors. The fulfilment of these inherent potentials is, however, dependent on the plasticity of the nervous system and post-birth experiences for their proper development.

The *plasticity of the nervous system* provides both the organic and functional bases for neuronal completion of the newborn infant's brain after birth. Plasticity, by affecting changes in the *resistance* of the neurons and their neural synaptic connectors to sensory excitations, is an essential factor in this *development of higher skills and behaviors* after birth. The plasticity of the neural synaptic connectors unites networks of dendritic and axodendritic nerve branches (arborizations), running between the billions of neurons within the brain. These connectors function as electronic gates controlling the great flow of neural sensations throughout the complex of neural networks, between and within the various levels of the brain.

This great flow of sensory excitations requires a *selection process* for monitoring the barrage on the neurons. This selection process is largely monitored by the complex differential biochemical transmissions of the neurons to their synaptic connectors in the form of neurotransmitters or neuroinhibitors. Each neuron is an extremely complex chemical factory manufacturing *neurotransmitters* and *neuroinhibitors*, which respectively permit or resist the flow of sensory excitations across the neuron's synaptic connectors. Each neuron is reported to have from 1000 to 10 000 synapses which receive sensory excitations from another 1000 interacting neurons.

The differential biochemical responses by the neurons vary in their potency to *permit or resist the passage of selective sensory excitations across the synaptic connectors*. These varying biochemical responses relate to the specific levels of synaptic *resistance*, which become *selectively preferential* to the sensory excitations transmitted by the perception systems and other multiple bodily sources. Neural plasticity, therefore, enables the neurons, and their synaptic connectors, to establish levels of resistance to compatible sensory excitations.

Reacting to the specific characteristics of the sensory excitations, the synaptic connectors may permit or inhibit their passage to neurons with specific functions. Each passage will therefore tend to *reinforce* the particular assemblies of neurons to sensory excitations *compatible* with their established levels of resistance, i.e. their preference. Plasticity also serves to protect the genetically specified neuronal functions in relation not only to the formation and performances of its multiple skills and behaviors, but also to the *development* and *maintenance* of the organism's life-support systems as well.

The importance of neural plasticity of the nervous systems to the organism's specific developmental and functional priorities was expressed by Moyer (1976):

> The synaptic connections, by virtue of their different levels of resistance to sensory excitations, tend to function as 'genetic controls'; selectively determining which neurons and their cell-assemblies, are to be preferentially activated.

Hebb (1949), within his neurophysiological approach to learning, stated that the hierarchy of preferential plasticity, coupled with the genetic specificity for primitive geometric forms, enabled young children to reproduce these forms imitatively without cognitive awareness of their meanings. Keele (1968) held that preferential plasticity also applied to neural cell assemblies with the genetic specificity for basic human skills, i.e. language, speech and reading. It would be unreasonable, he contended, considering the nervous system's graded chemical responses, not to apply neural plasticity to children's maturational, intellectual, emotional and motor developments.

Before children can develop particular skills, whether these are walking, speech, reading, etc., neural plasticity is necessary for the formation and automation (habituation) of the basic neurophysiological processes relative to the skill. Children can therefore vocally imitate echolalic and jargon patterns, formed as basic neurophysiological motor processes in their developing functional speech, rather than from cognitive comprehension of the meaning of these pre-speech vocalizations, which have yet to be developed.

Comments: we can observe, in neural plasticity, a rational basis for the *maturational transition* of the children's undifferentiated behaviors to more specifically goal-directed behaviors. It should be noted, however, that although neural plasticity serves in the automation of the neurophysiological perceptual–motor processes for specific skills, it may also promote the relative fixation of disturbed perceptual–motor skills and behaviors, such as *dyslexia* and *developmental stuttering*.

Brain development and neurophysiological functions related to the formation of basic skills

The neuropsychology of learning is based on the concept that external stimuli can effectively have a positive or negative influence on the neurophysiological functions of specific neural cell assemblies within the brain. A brief overview of some pertinent aspects of the brain may provide background insights into the functional bases for this concept.

The newly born infant, free of inherent, congenital or post-birth deficits, is a remarkably genetically designed and uniformly developing organism, composed of complex and interacting body systems that function with relative consistency towards harmonious maturation. The newly born infant has been regarded as a most dependent organism for a chronologically long period of time. Yet, within this grasping–groping infant lies the genetic potentials for highly sophisticated skills and behaviors awaiting the impetus of environmental stimuli to set them towards their remarkable developments.

The development of these skills and behaviors is made possible by a complex of interacting organizations of neurons and neural networks, referred to as the central nervous system. This unique mechanism provides the developing child with the capability to perceive, transmit, store, process, manipulate, collate, communicate, ideate, etc., vast amounts of information at fantastic speeds with relative consistency and reliability. The central nervous system unites the various bodily systems, which require proper nourishment and stimulation to assure their normal growth, maintenance and functional harmony. The central nervous system itself craves a constant diet of special compounds and sensory stimulations, especially during the child's early formative years. Rosenthal (1977) referred to the human nervous system as:

> . . . a very functional integrated central nervous system with complete association tracts, both within the cortex, and from the cortex to the deep brain areas.

During its evolutionary development, the brain expanded, resulting in a progressive increase in the distances between the individual brain cells (neurons) and a corresponding decrease in their density. As these billions of neurons moved apart from each other, the length and arborization (branches) of their interconnecting fibers, neural dendrites and axodendrites multiplied geometrically, affecting greater integration among the billions of neurons. These arborization processes, extremely active during the fetal stages, also continue during the child's early post-birth years (Rose, 1973).

The development of the human brain is regarded as comprising three main stages:

1. From conception to birth: the increase in brain size is mainly the result of the geometrical increase in the number of brain cells.
2. From birth to 12 months: continued increase in brain size is the result of:
   (a) on-going division of brain cells;
   (b) increase in the size of individual brain cells;
   (c) neural arborization (branching out).
3. From 12 months to maturity: the brain cells continue to grow in size, neural arborization occurs and there is increased myelination (the formation of insulation sheaths around the nerve fibers).

The great increase in numbers of brain cells, and arborization of billions of the interconnecting nerve fibers, resulted in the formation of the different levels and divisions of neuronal networks. Within each level, organizations of cell assemblies assumed different genetic specificities for particular skills and behaviors. In this regard, Moyer (1976) commented:

> . . . each brain level is comprised of general neuronal systems, which are so differentiated from each other in their genetic-specificity or the particular skills and behaviors, as to appear to function as – an entire unit.

There is, therefore, a hierarchy of neural influences between the various brain levels. This hierarchy relates to the extent to which neuronal systems at one level may influence the functions of neuronal systems within another brain level, or within the same level. This hierarchy is contingent upon such factors as:

- The multiplicity and complexity of the neuronal systems between each brain level, and within each level.
- The interactive connective associations of the neurons within the various neuronal systems, and between and within the various brain levels.
- The complexity of the genetically specified skill or behavior.
- The differential levels of synaptic resistance (plasticity) between the various neuronal systems.

As the various levels of the brain develop, their different functions become interrelated. These interrelationships enable the neuronal systems within each brain level to draw upon functions of other brain levels to complement the progressive formation of their particular genetically specified skills. Authorities have regarded the neurophysiological construct of the human brain as consisting of general and subgroup neuronal systems, contained within the several cortical levels and lower nerve centers. These neuronal systems are the following:

1. The general neuronal systems consist of the repositories for the multiple organizations of neurons (cell assemblies) within and between the various levels of the brain. These cell assemblies possess the genetic specificity for intellect, language–speech, writing, among other functional skills and behaviors.
2. The subgroup neurons are within the organizations of general neuronal systems, and function as triggering mechanisms for activating many types of neurons, including neurons with the genetic specificity for higher skills.
3. The subgroup neurons, as the result their natural lower neurosynaptic resistance, are prone initially to accept sensory excitations. This enables them to monitor transmission of excitation for preferential activation of particular organizations of neurons.

The perceptual–motor modalities are very responsive to external stimuli. The subgroup neurons are thus of special significance, because they are particularly responsive to the sensory excitations generated by the perceptual–motor modalities, namely, the visual, auditory and muscle systems. The significance of these relationships may be viewed as follows:

1. If the children's modes of perceptions are compatible with the basic

configurations of the objects being perceived, their sensory excitation subgroup neurons will reflect this compatibility, and transmit these excitations for passage to the specifically related general group neurons.
2. During the initial learning stages of a skill, such as reading, perceptual ambiguities may result in distorted modes of perceptions.

Such perceptions may, as a function of repetitions and neural plasticity, form disturbed neurophysiological processes within the organizations of neurons genetically specified for reading skill. These distorted perceptions may result in the disturbed neurophysiological processes becoming automated in the same manner as normal skill processes. Gerhardt related this to the difficulty in treating reading disorders

Comments: the above incompatible neural events would, I suggest, relate more particularly to functional behavioral disorders such as dyslexia than to other perceptual–motor disorders such as developmental stuttering. The logic of this contention is that children, more commonly having developed a functional degree of speech fluency before exhibiting stuttering behaviors, thus retain development of the basic neurophysiological motor–speech processes. Children, on the contrary, even though learning to read at a later maturational age, are more likely to exhibit reading disorders relative to their disturbed initial efforts to learn to read.

Gerhardt, in his studies of perceptual–motor disorders, referred to the limits to which one neuronal system may effect changes within other systems. These limits are the result of the resistance of genetically specific neurons to extreme changes. A child might incur extreme disorders in reading and yet the basic neurophysiological movements for the skill would rarely be lost completely. Rather, some basic remnant of the skill remains which may possibly be developed.

Similar findings have also been noted for people with various forms of aphasic disorders. This concurs with Gerhardt's concept on the selective effects of external stimuli on the executive program's influences on the formation of specific skills. Gerhardt stated: 'External influences could "selectively" affect the formation of specific skills, rather than constitute a "generalized disturbance" to the formation of a variety of skills.'

Neurophysiological conditions related to learning

Before Hebb, no theory on human behavior seemed to relate in specific human behaviors convincingly to individual neurons. Concerning this relationship, Hebb (1959) commented:

> To understand the on-going sensory interactions between the 'neuropsychological' components in the formation of a skill, requires relating 'physiology to psychology'.

Hebb considered the main problems with the theories on human behavior to be:

> For the physiologist: it was the problem of the transmission of sensory excitations from the perceptual modalities to the motor cortex within the brain.
> For the psychologist: it was the problem of human thought.

Although Hebb emphasized this dualistic approach to human behavior in early studies about learning, he did, however, tend to place greater stress on neurophysiological, rather than upon neuropsychological, factors. Although he attended more to the psychological aspects of learning in his later studies on children's development, there appeared to be certain limitations in his assertions on human behaviors.

We have noted that the infant's genetic specificity for the basic skills, i.e. language, speech, reading, writing, etc., are inherent potentials to be developed, rather than instinctive attributes. Such skills therefore require certain conditions for their proper development. These conditions, according to Fitts (1973), are also subject to the interactions between the neurogenic and neurophysiological components of the skill to be learned.

Hebb, however, closely related these interactions to the ability of young children to reproduce simple geometric forms imitatively; he used this as a basis for his neurophysiological approach to learning. He held this ability to be a genetically specified function of individual neurons; thus, the children need not understand the forms. He stated that:

> . . . unity and identity have separate 'neurophysiological' bases; with figural identity established 'only after' frequent repetitions of the configurations the child perceived and attempted to perform.

Hebb's neurophysiological approach to learning related more closely to the neurogenic than to the neuropsychological components. He held that, during the children's early stages of learning, their perceptual–motor performances reinforced their primitive genetic unity and identity experiences, rather than altering them. This does not conform with the findings of the Lurias about learned behaviors.

Hebb's neurophysiological conceptual system attempted to correlate the functions of individual neurons with specific psychological phenomena, i.e. the children's perceptual reproductions of the primitive forms. By asserting that individual neurons mainly accounted for the children's perceptions of simple specific configurations, he thus limited this system to its dependence on genetic specificity. He maintained that:

1. Neural cell assemblies are formed gradually during infancy, as a result of repeated specific sensory events.
2. Several neural cell assemblies, simultaneously and repeatedly activated, combine to form, along with their motor components, the 't' assembly. This assembly is regarded as corresponding to the perception of the distinctive events as a whole, i.e. the shape of a circle, a triangle, a square, etc.
3. Whereas neurons within the cell assemblies have motor cells, the child could perform his perceptions of these simple configurations without the need to understand them.

Hebb's conceptual system for learning, however, lead to his concepts on closed-loop memory tracks. These tracks contain the formation of neurophysiological perceptual–motor processes relative to the children's imitative performances of the drawings. These processes become progressively automated within these loops as motor programs, and thus prone to be repeated imitatively. His concepts about closed-loop memory tracts, within which the neurophysiological processes for the children's drawings become automated as motor programs, apparently provided Gerhardt with his novel insights into the neurophysiological formation of disturbed reading behaviors.

Neurophysiologically based motor programs

We might relate more accurately the importance of the concepts on motor programs to the neurophysiological formation of stuttering behaviors by Keele's (1968) description of motor programs as:

> . . . likened to 'internal blueprints', which consists of memory traces of the perceptual movements of the sensory modalities, and the subsequent 'perceptual-motor movements' activated by the responding neuronal systems.

Trumble and Noble (1973) regarded the motor program as critical to the formation of basic skills. They considered the motor program to be:

> . . . essential to the outflow of the sensory enervation, and the monitoring of the temporal-sequencing of the perceptual-motor movements required for the performance of a particular skill.

Fitts and Patterson (1964) defined motor programs as: the formation within a closed-loop tract of the temporal sequences of subroutine processes, which represent the distinct characteristics of the perceptual–motor movements relative to the neurophysiological motor performances of a particular skill. He commented further:

> As the skill develops, the 'sub-routines', representing portions of the total movement patterns of the intended skill, were seen to become more 'automated', and thus, more autonomous with respect to monitoring by the 'executive (master) program'.

The executive (master) program for speech and internal programs of action

The executive (master) program was considered by Fitts and Patterson (1964) to be: 'A sort of overall master-plan of the intended skill.'

The neuropsychological components of the executive (master) program mediate the neurophysiological components within the motor program for the skill. The motor program for the particular skill is therefore integrated within and subject to monitoring by the executive (master) program (Fitts and Patterson, 1964) The reader may note a similarity between Fitt's temporal sequences of subroutines, and Gerhardt's directional laterality of the modes of perception for neurophysiological processes formed within the motor program for the skill. Both refer to the perceptual–motor movements formed by the individual's perceptions of the tasks relative to the skill being learned.

Fitts considered that speech maintains its executive (master) program as does each specified skill. The executive (master) program for speech comprises the neurogenc, neurophysiological and neuropsychological components relative to speech skills. This program encompasses complexes of interacting neuronal networks within the cortical centers related to speech, such as the genetically specific neurons and motor cells, as well as the cognitive–perceptual systems, the muscle systems, intellect, memory and emotions, and related sentient responses, etc.

This program comprises, for example, the neuropsychological factors essential for affecting the transition of children's egocentric speech towards its use as a purposeful personal and social tool. The highly egocentric nature of young children is a basic neuropsychological variable that is important to their speech development. The children's highly self-centered need for gratification experiences greatly motivates their continued use of vocalizations as a ready means for satisfying their sentient appetites.

Rosenthal related young children's egocentric nature to their developing speech. He regarded speech as the most assertive of their early basic skills, and best suited for serving their egocentric behaviors. He considered their echolalic and babbling vocalizations to be the more obvious of their egocentric behaviors: 'The children's echolalic and babbling behaviors require little, if any, conscious thought with regard to their application as a functional, let alone a "social tool".'

> These early 'egocentric vocalizations' characterize the children's 'genetic specificity' for speech. They also provide the 'perceptual–motor movements' and stimulations necessary for preparing the neurophysiologic bases for speech development.

Rosenthal further contended that children's egocentric, self-stimulating vocalizations, babbling and echolalic speech were indicative of their earliest consistent perceptions of certain speech patterns. This early conscious awareness of vocal–language relationships is the result of the influences of the children's expanding and stimulating socioenvironments, within which they seek increasing human contacts. The children's early social experiences thus serve to promote the transition of the children's egocentric speech towards its functional use through the overall controlling mediation of an executive (master) program for speech.

The neuropsychological components, particularly the cognitive–perceptual and emotional faculties, are particularly sensitive to environmental influences. These faculties are also regarded effectively to influence each other during the transition of the child's early developing speech into a social tool. This transition does not necessarily mean removal of the egocentricity as a major factor in development of the child's speech skills. On the contrary, this transition usually constitutes, more or less, an orderly transference from the child's egocentric speech for self-gratification to its conformity to social influences.

It is one thing for the child to obtain gratification by his use of early speech. It is, however, quite another thing to do so by intentionally changing his speech performances to meet external demands/standards; the child may not properly perceive, let alone understand, this. To do so requires the functions of an executive (master) program, dependent on internal programs of action. These internal programs are speech experiences, which enable the child to act upon cognitive perceptions of his past performances to selectively perform the necessary changes perceived to be required (Cole, 1978).

Cole maintained that to act with volition is to internalize cognitive perceptions and experiences. He considered that without such internalization: '. . . the neuronal processes would only be associated with purely imitative performances.' Cole was referring to functions within the young child's higher cortical neuronal centers, which integrate information and prior experiences pertaining to the particular skill. The formation of internal programs for action is a function of a conglomerate of neurons, located within the frontal lobes of the brain, which are considered to contain the neuronal centers for integrating information from both sides of the brain, as well as for acting with volition.

> *Comments*: this attention to the executive (master) program will be shown, within the following chapters, to be particularly pertinent to stuttering, because it serves, by virtue of its neuropsychological components, as the central mediator in a stutterer's repeated involuntary episodes of stuttering behaviors, and the resistance of these behaviors to therapy methods.

Dyslexia and stuttering behaviors: bases for comparative neurophysiological similarities

> It is a general observation that there is a connection between stuttering, word-blindness (dyslexia), and handedness. The nature of this connection is not too well understood.
>
> *Gerhardt (1977)*

Humans are regarded to have communicated by oral means centuries before Guttenburg's printing press, and the complexities of maintaining large mercantile societies brought the need and the luxury of reading to the general public. This would suggest that humans exhibited stuttering behaviors long before reading disorders. Gerhardt does not, however, consider that the later development of reading skills or reading disorders negates his contentions of possible connections between dyslexia and stuttering. There is, however, insufficient research evidence to allude to etiological (causal) connections between reading disorders and stuttering.

There are, however, as Gerhardt (1977) contends, certain comparisons between reading and speech, which suggest possible neurophysiological similarities with regard to the neurophysiological processes relative to both: the normal, as well as the disruptive, formation of these two basic communicative skills. Some of the more dominant similarities between dyslexia and stuttering listed below can also apply to other types of behavioral disorders:

- Each disorder relates disturbances to a genetically specific communication skill.
- Both disorders can relate to disturbing perceptions of external stimuli.
- Both disorders are regarded to evidence perceptual–motor disturbances involving the sensory and motor systems.
- Both reading and speech use symbols: graphic and phonetic (sound) respectively.

- Both disorders can occur in individuals with no known evidence of prior inherent, congenital or post-birth anomalies. Depending on one's perspective, this point may be subject to disagreement, in spite of the lack of contradictory evidence.
- Both exhibit involuntary performances related to disturbed neurophysiological perceptual–motor processes.
- Both tend to lead to relative states of emotional disturbance, which may lead to more severe neuropsychological consequences.
- Both may lead to the use of and preoccupation with coping adjustment methods.
- Both may lead to negative anticipations relating to the outcome of their intended performances.
- Both have shown relatively consistent stubborn resistance to a variety of remedial techniques.
- Both disorders are regarded as relating to a wide variety of different etiologies.

Comments: the above similarities between dyslexia and stuttering do not necessarily confirm etiological (causal) connections between them. The only possible connection, however, may, as noted earlier, be in the relative similarities in the effects of disturbing perceptual influences on neuronal events, leading to the disturbed neurophysiological motor processes respective to each disorder.

Chapter 2
The neurophysiology of dyslexia

Introduction

This discussion on dyslexia in no way suggests any causal (etiological) relationships between writing disorders and stuttering behaviors. It is intended only to support the notion that comparative similarities exist, not only in the neuronal formation of the basic neurophysiological motor processes for the development and performances of perceptual–motor skills, be it walking, writing, speech, etc. (defined by Fitts, 1966), but also with regard to the formation of particular disorders relative to perceptual–motor skills (Gerhardt, 1977).

Consistent with the above notion, this book endeavors rationally to apply what is known about the disturbed neurophysiological motor processes for reading disorders towards gaining a better understanding of the lesser known factors that lead to the neuronal formation and sustainment of stuttering behaviors.

Aristotle stated, 'Knowledge to be learned, must first be perceived by the senses'. Developing basic skills therefore depends on proper perceptual–motor movements, which are essential for all sensory perceptions: visual, auditory, tactile and proprioceptive. Movements are basic to the experiences the child needs for learning.

Hebb (1949), in discussion of the importance of movements, commented:

> Movement effectively influences the 'neurophysiological' bases for the organization and activation of the neural networks within the human nervous system, and in particular, within the higher cortical levels of the brain.

Although it is quite evident that proper movements are essential for writing and speech performances, it might surprise many to learn that movements are fundamental to the development of the proper neurophysiological motor processes for competent reading skills.

Gerhardt (1977) referred to the child's dependence on perceptual–motor movements for developing reading skills as follows:

> Learning is a chain of production with each link a process smoothly integrated with a preceding and subsequent process; and the key to the stable flow of events along this chain – is movement.

Definitions and projected causes for dyslexias

Dyslexia relates to reading disabilities which are generally defined in broad terms. Perhaps, this may to be the result of the lack of a consensus with regard to their etiological perspectives. To cite a few examples:

> Dyslexia is:
>
> Commonly used to identify children with reading difficulties, and often associated with the term 'word-blindness'.
>
> *Gerhardt (1977)*
>
> A reading difficulty of indeterminable etiology.
>
> *Kolb and Whishaw (1980)*
>
> Often used when neurological dysfunction is suspected as the cause for the child's reading difficulties.
>
> *Naidoo (1972)*
>
> Frequently used to refer to a condition causing those afflicted to have extreme difficulty in acquiring reading skills. It simply means an inability to read.
>
> *Lerner (1985)*

Lerner (1985) listed the more currently held causes for reading (dyslexic) disturbances as being indicative of:

1. Evidence of brain disorders.
2. Genetic factors.
3. Syndrome of maturational lag.
4. Behavioral manifestation of central nervous system dysfunction.
5. Synonym for reading retardation.

Lerner thought that the literature on dyslexia could be categorized along two main lines of thought, each based on its own distinctive perspective:

1. The medical perspective: dyslexia is the result of an inability to read caused by brain damage or central nervous system dysfunction.
2. The educational perspective: dyslexia is indicative of something

wrong with a child's reading, as a consequence of disturbed learning skills, and better than average or highly intelligent children finding it difficult to read.

(For a further listing of the multiple definitions and causes projected for reading disorders, see Appendix II.)

In summary dyslexia, as noted above and in Appendix II, has been attributed to an extremely diverse assortment of singular and multiple causes, which is indicative of an apparent lack of any consistent etiological perspective. In Chapter 3, a similar extensive listing of etiological assertions is listed for stuttering, which led Gerhardt to state:

> One problem is that both stuttering and dyslexia are single names of multiple states which should be differentiated.

(For additional causes and definitions for dyslexia, see Appendix I.)

Incidence of dyslexia in American and Japanese schoolchildren

The high incidence of dyslexia (reading incompetence) among schoolchildren is a major national problem. Studies of large populations of American schoolchildren have reported incidences of reading disabilities, ranging from 16 to 20%. These incidences excluded variations in test results related to ethnic, geographical and socioeconomic factors. When the lowest reported incidence of 10% is equated with the approximately 6 million American schoolchildren, an awesome minimum of at least 600 000 children are in need of remedial reading programs.

In 1968, Kiyoski Makita, Professor of Neuropsychiatry and Director of Children's Psychiatric Services at Keio University of Medicine, published a report comparing the incidence of dyslexia among Japanese schoolchildren and those of Western nations, in particular the USA. Dr Makita reported that, of 9195 Japanese schoolchildren surveyed, less than 1% were regarded as having exhibited reading difficulties. Allowing for the mentally handicapped students, the percentage was considered to be 0.89–0.98%. Makita related these differences to the distinct cultural differences between Japanese and the Western languages, namely the Kana and the Roman alphabets.

Makita stated further:

1. These significant high incidences of reading disabilities could not be due to inherent, congenital, or post-birth pathologies, but rather to external factors.

2. The greater numbers of the Western schoolchildren exhibiting reading disabilities were developing normally prior to their incurring reading disabilities.

The Japanese Kana and the Roman alphabet (see Appendix II)

Makita contended that the Roman alphabet, common to the languages of Western nations, contains ambiguous script–phonetic relationships which could account for the disturbing perceptions of the alphabet among their schoolchildren. Makita stressed his conviction by stating:

> Theories which ascribe the etiology of reading disability to localized cerebral abnormalities to laterality conflict, or to emotional pressure, may be valid in some instances, but the specificity of the used language is the most potent factor in the formation of reading disability.

Rosenthal (1977) referred to the inconsistencies and ambiguities of the English (Roman) alphabet's script–phonetic relationships as follows:

> English is phonetic in the sense that separate sounds of the language are represented graphically by printed symbols.
>
> In English, there are forty-eight phonemes, of which seventeen are vowels, and thirty-one are consonants. The forty-eight phonemes are represented by only twenty-six letters or combinations of letters.
>
> Therefore, the phoneme-to-phoneme association in English is not fully systematic; some would say that it is confused and therefore, it is said that the 'orthography' of the English language is highly irregular.

The neurophysiology of dyslexia

This section is concerned only with depicting the potentials of ambiguous external stimuli to disturb children's perceptual–motor systems, through the imposition of disturbing influences on the neurophysiological motor functions of neurons, with the genetic specificity for basic reading skills. The external ambiguities of the Roman alphabet's script–phonetic relationships were considered to be the primary external factors contributing to the high incidences of reading disorders among children regarded as normal.

The potential of disturbing perceptions of external stimuli was studied by Lund (Fitts, 1973), who reported on the neurophysiological effects of external stimuli on visual and auditory responsiveness in normal animals. He studied the directional selectivity of ocular nerve cells firing in response to specific forms of external stimuli. His findings showed that external stimuli disturbed the animals' sensory perceptions (modes of perception), affected the status, as well as the activation, of neurons within the visual cortex of their brains. He reported:

> . . . profound deficits in visual–motor control may be produced by disassociating visual and sensory feedback systems in the presence of perfectly normal vision.
>
> In the cerebral cortex, there were pronounced physiological aberrations. Although anatomical changes have been identified, they are more subtle and have been given perhaps less attention than they deserve.
>
> The main physiological affects of biocular deprivation are the reduction (or loss) of specifically responsive cells which respond sluggishly, are poorly tuned, or are unresponsive to visual stimuli. In the lateral geniculate nucleus, there is evidence of cell shrinkage at least throughout the laminae. There is good indication in the auditory system that comparable events may occur.

Although not producing such severe disturbing effects, the perceptual ambiguities of the script–phonetic relationships within the Roman alphabet presents functional difficulties to which the child's perceptual–motor modalities apparently cannot adapt readily. This presents distorted configurations, in the form of sensory excitations, transmitted to the visual–motor neurons within the brain. As with a camera, if the external conditions for taking photographs are inappropriate, the processed prints will be affected in spite of the proper working of the camera.

There is a fundamental difference, however, between the functional operation of the camera and the child's visual–perceptual modalities. The functions of the camera will not be affected, no matter how many poor prints are taken, whereas subjecting the child's visual modalities to repeated disturbing stimuli, such as the ambiguous script–phonetic relationships, will affect his normal perceptual–motor functions.

Furthermore, unlike the camera, what the child perceives must be understood to be properly acted upon. The disturbed perceptions of the Roman alphabet affect disruptive changes in the formation of the neurophysiological motor processes or reading, which, as a result of neural plasticity, become chronic dyslexic behaviors. Fitts, and Hebb, emphasized the importance of the neurophysiological motor processes within closed-circuit motor programs as basic to learning reading skills.

In addition, the child who cannot perceive and imitate the basic characteristics of the Roman alphabet is deprived of gratifying experiences which can motivate repetition of his imitative efforts. This can lead to confusion and negative emotional states, which, in turn, can affect the child's neuronal centers for reading. Their continued efforts to perform the basic reading tasks become more uncertain, and less gratifying. Whereas other children have begun reading to learn, they are still attempting to learn to read.

Dyslexic disabilities, as with stuttering behaviors, can have severe emotional and social consequences as Naidoo (1972) expressed:

> Lack or incompetency in reading and writing can lead to disaster for an individual in a society whose intricacies and successes are based upon the 'graphic-symbol' interpretation.
>
> Employability is increasing contingent upon literacy. Those who cannot read today are to be the 'disadvantaged' of tomorrow. They may well be impoverished economically and emotionally, and their misfortune may be felt in various ways; by their families, and by the society in which they live.

Comments: at the risk of being redundant, this discussion on dyslexia is intended only to depict the potential of disturbing perceptions of external stimuli for disrupting neurophysiological motor performances of a genetically specified skill such as reading. As a result of the similarities between reading and speech, it is contended that neurophysiological motor processes for speech can also be disrupted by disturbing perceptions of external stimuli, as is evident in stuttering behaviors, which can result in consequences comparable to those above described by Naidoo.

Chapter 3
Overview of the symptoms, theories, definitions and psychosocial factors relevant to developmental stuttering

Developmental stuttering: a unique human behavioral disorder

This chapter will touch upon topics that are discussed in greater detail later in the book. These topics, likened to clues in a complex puzzle, will provide the readers with insight into the need for a more comprehensive understanding of stutterering and stutterers, and for realistic approaches to treatment with therapy and to psychosocial problems.

From only a cursory reading of the literature, it becomes apparent that stuttering is commonly regarded as a most complex form of human behavioral disorder. We might question, however, how much of this general impression is the result of multiple layers of speculative theorization, contradictions and misconceptions, which have, over many years, contributed greatly to this perplexing impression.

The basic cause(s) for stuttering is still considered to be unknown. Much has been written, however, about the multiple factors that influence the production of its diverse range of symptoms and associated behaviors. Yet, proper treatment of stuttering remains limited and inconsistent. In this regard, it seems strange that there has been relatively little study of the extent to which neuropsychological and psychosocial factors contribute, not only towards its formative development, or the repeated episodes of stutterering behaviors, but also to the apparent resistance of these behaviors to therapy methods.

Many authorities agree that undue external stimuli on the child's speech efforts can promote negative conditions, which influence the transition of early non-fluencies towards dysfluency behaviors. Little attention has been given to these external factors that promote this transition, and the subsequent formation of developmental stuttering. External influences, such as personal or group standards and biases, often determine which individuals are accorded the appropriate opportunities for pursuing talents and vocational aspirations. There have been historical periods during which stutterers were judged to be possessed by devils, to be mentally incompetent or to have severe mental illness; they were treated accordingly.

Within our more modern, sophisticated societies, such views are deemed archaic to our advanced knowledge of human behaviors and our enlightened views about human dignity. Stutterers may no longer be burned, flogged or confined, but they are often regarded with tolerant indifference. Although many stutterers do achieve success, many others, as noted earlier, are disadvantaged. They must often compromise social and/or vocational needs for a modicum of submissive security on the fringe of the public mainstream. This, in no small part, is the result of the misconceptions of the general public, which are sometimes professionally promoted and which lead to negative personal and family consequences comparable to those Naidoo described for dyslexic subjects.

Speech: a too highly valued commodity?

> Of all the singular gifts bestowed on human beings, the ability to speak is perhaps the most miraculous, and the most taken for granted. Children are expected to begin to talk intelligibly almost before they are out of swaddling clothes; if they don't, their way-wardness is a cause of valid concern.
>
> Newsweek (*1986*)

The above expresses general parental expectancies and anxieties, often foisted upon young children, to develop good speech. Children, however, differ in maturation and exposure to environmental stimuli. Such factors tend to be forgotten when speech alone is used as a measure of the child's maturational development, and as the criterion for determining normal development. Speech skills, within our highly technotronic society, are a highly valued and much sought commodity for enhancing personal, social and vocational successes (Mandell, 1983). Pretentious speech skills have become an all too common ploy for creating illusions without substance; a façade for success within the political, corporate and professional sectors (Toffler, 1970).

Many normal speakers with aspiring ambitions thus seek the services of voice and speech–language therapists. This growing trend is subject to serious question when the means to communicate become more highly valued than the message, although many in need of speech and language therapy find such services unavailable or too costly. The objectives for changing speech skills become suspect when intended mainly for fostering illusions of competence, trust and intelligence, so a jackass can sound like a thoroughbred. The above *Newsweek* article also reported that one of the first services employed by aspiring or newly elected politicians was the skills of voice or speech–language therapists.

Good speech is a valid objective, but demands for pretentious speech can impose unrealistic pressures on young students to meet such deceptive standards for success. The negative behaviors may result from the stress-provoking, although well-meaning, emphasis parents, teachers or others place on children's speech. Such undue emphasis can lead to serious psychosocial problems for the child, the parents and, subsequently, the community. One such problem may be developmental stuttering.

Increased emphasis on affected speech skills has promoted the extensive increase in university and college speech and language training and clinic programs, as well as private clinic programs, which have shown considerable profit potentials. Still, there is an acknowledged shortage of speech pathologists to treat the more than 10 million Americans, mostly children, in need of speech and language therapy (*Newsweek*, 1980). To what extent does this over-emphasis to affect speech skills contribute to the apparent growth in related behavioral problems, such as stuttering?

Speech, from its earliest onset, provides a kind of wireless umbilical unity for the young infant and his parents, enabling them to interact intimately at ever-increasing distances. Speech is the young child's most natural, versatile and readily available medium for communication. Chomsky (1965) regarded the young child's potential to develop speech and language as:

> . . . humans have a biological basis for developing language skills, which are inherently determinable.

Speech enables the young child to establish and express self-object relationships, which are basic for acquiring language and cognitive skills. Speech is also essential for the child's development of self-assertiveness, which will affect his current and future developments greatly (Rosenthal, 1977).

> *Comments*: speech pathologists strongly advise that, with proper care and affection within stimulating and pleasurable speech environments, children will develop competent speech sufficient to meet their social and vocational needs. This offers a far better alternative than causing children to become confused, frustrated and later possibly disadvantaged because of ill-advised concerns and attentions for pretentious speech standards.

Symptoms and deficits attributed to stuttering

In science, one gets such wholesome returns of conjecture out of such a trifling investment of fact.

Mark Twain

Our knowledge of stuttering has been obtained primarily from observing its occurrences and characteristics within both applied and speculative research. Below is a compendium of some of the widely diverse, inherent or acquired deficits and symptomatologies reported in research on stuttering over the last 60 years or so:

Stutterers show a significantly lower 'pH' in their saliva.

Kelly (1932)

Stutterers exhibit disturbed perceptions of visual symbols, with marked lower performances on visual aphasic tests.

Kelly (1932)

Stutterers show marked differences in the EMG reading for the masseter muscles bilaterally during stuttering.

Travis (1934)

Stutterers perform like the ambidextrous group on the Critical Angle Board.

Van Riper (1935)

Stutterers perseverate more than normals on a motor test.

Eisenson and Pastel (1938)

Stutterers show neural dys-synchrony during speech in the activity brain waves within the two hemispheres of the brain.

Travis and Knott (1937)

Stutterers have a faster heart rate prior to speech than normals.

Travis, Tuttle and Cowan (1936)
Palmer and Gillette (1939)

Emotional imbalances: stutterers are more neurotic, introverted, and less confident, and dominant than non-stutterers.

Bender (1938)

There is no difference between stutterers and controls in pH.

Hafford (1941)

General bodily incoordinations: stutterers are poorer than non-stutterers in rhythm and coordinations tests.

Strother and Kreigman (1944)

Hostility: stuttering as a consequence of desire to avoid speech which is regarded to constitute an act of hostility.

Fenichel (1945)

There is little, if any, stuttering in primitive cultures.

Bullen (1945)

Prevalence of stuttering in twins: 13% incidence.

Nelson, Hunter and Walter (1945)

When primitive cultures are under pressure, they tend to show increased stuttering, as does placing people in a university which causes them to stutter more than the average population

Lemert (1953)
Schuell (1946)

Motor retardation: in stuttering children ranging from two to five years.

Kopp (1946)

Anal fixation.

Dickson (1946)

Lower intelligence.

Schindler (1955)

Mental retardation.

Schlanger and Gottsleben (1957)

Stuttering is related to epilepsy, particularly to pyknolepsy.

West (1958)

Between two and five times more males than females stutter.

West (1958)
Berry and Eisenson (1956)
Van Riper and Emerick (1984)

Seizure predisposition: stuttering is a compulsive disorder akin to epilepsy (epileptiform) form in childhood.

West (1958)

Psychosexual fixations: stuttering as covert evidence of infantile libidinous and repressed pregenital sexuality.

Glauber (1958)

Approach-avoidance conflict: stuttering due to conflicts in child's wish to speak and not speak.

Sheehan (1970)

Stuttering children have poorer sound localization than normals.

Rousey, Goetzinger and Dirks (1959)

Stutterers show higher levels of alpha waves.

Shopwin (1959)

Dichotic lag: results in degradation of auditory (verbal) stimuli found due to left ear preference in stutterers.

Kimura (1973)

Stutterers and normals perform the same with regard to perseveration on motor test.

Martin (1962)

Stutterers prefer cool colors in their water color paintings as compared to normals.

Laczkowska (1965)

Cortical blood flow: higher in Broca's area on right side during stuttering, in Wernicke's area on left.

Shrum (1984)

Biochemical imbalances: metabolic and chemical differences disrupt neurophysiological mechanisms for speech.

West (1958)

GSR response to stimuli is delayed in stutterers as opposed to normals.

Dinnan, McGuiness and Perrin (1970)

Neurogenic stuttering: due to damage to the nervous system.

Canter (1981)

Down's syndrome: 34% of 48 stutterers.

Preus (1972)

Cerebral dominance: greater preference for left hemisphere processing of verbal stimuli.

Moore and Haynes (1980)

Genetic traits: gene–environment interaction to be high predictor of inherent stuttering.

Kidd (1977)

Muscle incoordinations: laryngeal muscles disrupt speech processes resulting in physiological blocks.

Freeman and Ushijima (1978)

Depressed alpha rhythms over right posterior-parietal area; accounting for significantly shorter attention span.

Craven, Faber and Moore (1982)

Patilla and Achilles tendon reflexes become increased in stutterers.

Travis and Fagan (1928)

Touch and kinaesthetic insensitivity in right and left extremities.

Markham (985)

Conditioning processes as a primary cause for stuttering; laryngeal fixation.

Schwartz (1986)

All the above strongly suggest a compulsive hunt for symptoms and deficit behaviors to attribute to stuttering; unfortunately this has led to considerable misunderstanding about stuttering and misconceptions about stutterers. This multiplicity of symptoms and deficit behaviors would tend to depict stutterers as akin to some form of unearthly multipathologically disturbed mutation residing in our midst in the guise of an apparently normal-looking human.

> *Comments*: when such questionable research findings represent professional views towards stuttering and stutterers, what might be the general public's attitudes and responses towards stutterers? Considering the absurd array of symptoms and behavioral deficits and symptoms reported, it would at best appear most tolerant of the general public to respond to them with benign indifference, rather than, as in the past, subject them to superstitions, abuse, denigations, confinements, etc.

It is deemed to be worth while repeating Bloodstein's (1975) concerns regarding this ever-growing compendium of questionable symptoms and behavioral deficits:

> Can the 'typical stutterer' be depicted to be: anally fixated, brain-damaged with atypical cortical dominance, inadequate of sound-mindedness; to possess inter-aural-phase disparities, lower auditory pain thresholds, vascular and biochemical imbalances, and/or a multiple of other differential anomalies?

Theoretical approaches to stuttering

Stuttering has long been pursued by professionals, lay people and pseudoprofessionals who hope to legitimize their favorite theories and speculations. Although some have received more attention than others, none has managed consistently to maintain a dominant role on the center stage.

The listing below of some past and current and theoretical approaches indicates some of the efforts of concerned professionals to use available knowledge, and their own experiences, towards a better understanding of stuttering, and to provide more beneficial and consistent therapy.

Mechanical theory

In the past, it has been suggested that stuttering may be caused by faulty breathing, enlarged tonsils, or even by extensive vegetative growth of the adenoids.

Environmental theory

Stuttering may be caused by distressing environmental conditions:

1. Horrible living conditions. Very poor diets.
2. Constant problems within the home.
3. Punitive attitudes and treatments towards the child, evoking fear of speaking because of uncertainty about the responses that may ensue.

Advocates of these, and related, theories generally regarded individuals, before they started to stutter, as having been constitutionally and psychologically no different from normally developing or developed speakers (Ainsworth, 1945).

Anxiety theories

Stuttering is regarded as a 'learned anxiety reaction system', and paradoxically reduction of anxiety may reinforce stuttering behaviors (Wischner, 1950).

Wischner noted a somewhat comparative analogy between stuttering behaviors from conditioning and those from learning experiments. He regarded the adaptation effect to be similar to experimental extinction, because if stuttering is to occur, a withdrawal of reinforcements is needed. He noted, however, that it is very difficult to identify the analogy mechanisms operating in stuttering behaviors.

Psychic theories

Stuttering may be the result of traumatic fright, shock or extreme remorse, and even high fever. Also, it may relate to supersensory or extrasensory mental functions of the human mind and soul, which, when disturbed, can result in 'psychic stuttering' (Feiderman, 1951).

Traumatic theories

Stuttering is caused by extreme nervous reactions to traumatic experiences, often characterized by uneasiness or apprehension. Traumatic experiences may be related to either a mother being frightened during prenatal period or stresses and strains associated with important personal/social situations.

These are among the oldest theories for stuttering. They assume that stresses and strains during certain anxiety situations tend to clutter the person's thoughts, inducing mental hurriedness and also marked emotional changes. There are constitutional bases for these reactions which may be inherited or acquired by analogy.

Cultural theories

Stuttering results from early cultural pressures on the young child to exhibit standards of linguistic competences.

The onset of stuttering is deemed to be more or less gradual, resulting from the progressively sustained, conscious or unconscious, parental pressures on the children to master advanced conversational phrases and sentences.

Learned behavior theories

Stuttering is a learned behavior growing out of children's early non-fluency phase. They are able to express themselves, but tend to be unaware of exhibiting primary non-fluencies.

These children might, therefore, be subjected to undue parental concerns or coercions, in the form of ridicule or punishments, for not conforming to standards of speech they might not even comprehend. Learned behavior theories usually maintain that children's speech environments may have excessively negative influences which can effectively constitute fluency disruptors (Eisenson and Ogilvie, 1957). As stuttering is considered to be a learned behavior, it may respond to desensitization, i.e. unlearning remedial methods (Brutten and Shoemaker, 1967).

Stimulus generalization theories

Stuttering is attributed to sensitivity to particular words and/or situations, which may not have previously elicited dysfluency behaviors. This is the result of their association with certain traumatic experiences, which serve as triggering stimuli for stuttering behaviors (Peters and Simonson, 1960).

Neurotic theories

Stuttering is a symptom of a psychoneurotic condition, seen as an 'attention-getting device', i.e. a symptom of an inferiority complex.

It is also regarded as a symptom growing out of another less obvious, but effectively disturbing, problem; when this is removed the stuttering will disappear (Travis, 1957). Within the context of psychoneurosis, stuttering involves behaviors that indicate emotional maladjustments. Stuttering reflects the individual's inability to make a satisfactory social–speech adjustment to another person.

Neurotic theories have been one of the most dominant and long-held theories on stuttering. Disturbing influences of the misconceptions related to these theories still predominate among the public, and even the professional sectors.

Operant–behavioral theories

These theories do not directly specify singular or group causes for stuttering. Rather, stuttering is regarded as a behavior overtly responsive to the controling influences of reinforcing and often disagreeable environmental events (stimuli).

These theories imply conditioned conflicts between the physiological limitations of the organs of speech, and their more primary or genetically specified biological functions (Shames and Sherrick, 1963).

Approach-avoidance conflict theories

Stuttering is the ambivalent by-product of a conflict in decision-making. The child is burdened by guilt feelings for his early onset of stuttering behaviors, and experiences conflicting needs to express himself.

The child, within a particular situation, may feel the need to 'be silent and yet, not to be silent'. Stuttering represents a child's compromise between a need to speak and a need, out of guilt, to remain silent. Here, both the cause and its overt intensification in stuttering behaviors lie in guilt feelings (Sheehan, 1970).

Conflict-reinforcement theories

Stuttering symptoms represent behavioral expressions of conflicts in the interpersonal relationships between the child's sensory–perceptual systems and negative environmental influences.

Interpersonal communication theories

Stuttering is primarily a form of learned behavior, which occurs in response to anxieties. Anxieties are precipitated and reinforced by distorted perceptions of interpersonal relationships.

Therapy methods tend to focus mainly on establishing positive client–clinician relationships designed to provide a basis for manipulating the stutterer's identification processes – confrontation and introspection – for transference within his interpersonal relationships outside the clinical setting (Cooper, 1968)

Two-factor theories

Stuttering is the composite product of disturbing interplay between the child's genetic and environmental components for speech. The extent of this disturbance can determine the severity of the individual's stuttering behaviors.

Although implied in other theories for stuttering, the two-factor theory attempts a holistic approach to understanding and treating stuttering. Its main approach is to attempt to distinguish between the effective participation of the stutterer's involuntary and voluntary behaviors (Shames and Rubin, 1986).

These theories attempted to treat what are regarded as the symptomatic effects of involuntary genetic and environmental influences on the outcome of the individual's stuttering behaviors, such as the individual's volitional attempts to cope, in the form of 'speech-related struggles', with his stuttering behaviors (Shames and Rubin, 1986).

In summary the above listing of theories for stuttering is not conclusive. Little would be gained by attempting to list the larger number of theories historically projected. There has been and continues to be valued differences of opinions expressed as theories for stuttering. We may therefore also anticipate diverse differences in the definitions for stuttering presented within the next section.

Stuttering: in need of a practical definition

> A word is to mean, what I choose it to mean.
>
> *Lewis Carroll*

A proper definition should contain the basic characteristics and basic functions of that which it proposes to identify. It is therefore a matter of determining what and how much it should contain, if the definition is to be comprehensive and concise. A proper definition should be likened to what has been said of a bikini: 'which should sufficiently cover what need be, but not overly to dispel interest'.

Definitions for stuttering have long been subjected to extensive speculations, omissions, additions and contradictions. Stuttering is somewhat of a paradox in that, although relatively easy to identify, it has proved extremely difficult to define. Attempts to define stuttering have depended largely on observations and consensus agreements about its symptomatic behaviors. Some of these definitions are listed below:

1. Visual and/or auditory manifestations of tonic and/or clonic blockages to oral and/or laryngeal mechanisms.
2. Perceptual–motor or sensory modality disturbances resulting from neurophysiological factors.
3. Involuntary subjugation to powerful undercurrents of varying states of emotional to psychoneurotic manifestations: anxieties, aggression, passivity, guilt, maladjustments, etc.
4. Difficulty with word-finding and sentence formation.
5. Conditionally learned behavioral responses to negative stimuli.
6. Anticipatory anxiety responses in efforts to avoid or escape the occurrences of stuttering behaviors.
7. Hereditary familial characteristics of dysfluency behaviors.
8. Traumatic responses to anxiety-evoking experiences.

Historical overview of descriptive definitions for stuttering

A rose is a rose, is a rose.

G. Stein

Descriptive definitions for stuttering have tended to follow the erratic trends of prevailing research, schools of thought, professional biases, popularized gurus or other transient influences. Descriptive definitions for stuttering have therefore often assumed the chameleon-like characteristic of the mythical horse of a different color, as noted below:

1. Stuttering is a regressive fixation of the young child's anal tendencies to the oral level; providing oral pleasures (Brown, 1938).
2. Stuttering is a reversal in the child's speech processes in the effort to speak. He tries to say words rather than express thoughts (Hendricks, 1929).
3. Stuttering behavior manifests one of the few psychoneuroses starting in very early childhood and remains in the same form during adulthood. The stutterer does not want to spit out words, but the words become real objects.
4. Stuttering: is a symptom, an effect, not a cause. It is a symptom of emotional maladjustment, which is predisposing and exciting as a cause (Fisher, 1932).

   Fisher further stated: 'Without these emotional reaction tendencies, I believe stuttering would be impossible. The "drainage theory" enters here. The child's pent-up fears tries to find an outlet through the speech mechanism, and in doing so interferes with speech; usually resulting in partial paralysis of the speech muscles.'

5. The symptoms for stuttering usually arise during the ages of 3–8 years, and generally express such feelings as:
   (a) timidity;
   (b) insecurity;
   (c) inferiority;
   (d) fear with respect to others, particularly people in authority (Brown, 1945).
6. Stuttering behaviors: a vocal sign of infantile speech caused by a discrepancy between the young child's motor ability, and his rate of thinking (Davis, 1939).
7. Stuttering is defined as fluency difficulties manifesting clonic and tonic interruptions (Bryngelson, 1952).
8. Stuttering: frequent non-fluencies, and related behaviors, which society judges to call undue attention to a person's manner of speech and markedly interferes with communication, are to be regarded as stuttering (Ainsworth, 1945).

   Dr Ainsworth added a novel and subjective criterion for defining stuttering. She considered the symptoms for stuttering to be of minor importance. Of greater importance is the listener's judgment and tolerance of the person's need and ability to communicate. Ainsworth's practical definition for stuttering was typical of her humanist concerns for the public, as well as the clinical treatment of stutterers. As a former student of Dr Ainsworth, this book reflects the lasting impression of her excellent teaching.
9. Stuttering: a chronic extension of the child's normally developing speech patterns caused by disruptions to his neurophysiological motor processes for speech (Van Riper, 1954).

   Van Riper's neurophysiological approach to stuttering was in opposition to most of the prevailing approaches to stuttering, with his reference to primary stuttering as part of the child's 'normally developing speech'. He maintained that normal children could develop stuttering as a result of improper external (parental, etc.) influences upon their speech.
10. Stuttering is a condition formed from the child's perception of himself as a stutterer. This semantic-based perception is regarded as resulting from the unwarranted influences of his parents and others, which evokes inner awareness of confusion, anxieties and negative attitudes towards speech. He also referred to stuttering as 'lalaphonia' (Johnson, 1959).

    Johnson, like Van Riper, stressed the effectiveness of parental influences on the young child's developing speech. His major emphasis was, however, more upon the child's perceptions of himself and his speech than reactions to the perceptions of others.

    Johnson related his semantic concepts to stuttering, in which he embodied his definitions. In spite of his claim to a parapsychological approach, his remedial methods appeared to be similar to Van Riper's basic neurophysiological approach. Johnson regarded his approach to be a semantically based diagnostogenic concept for stuttering.

11. Stuttering and associative behaviors are to be defined in terms of 'constitutional predisposition factors' (Bluemel, 1960).

    Bluemel contended that many children are constitutionally predisposed to develop stuttering, but do not do so because, like allergies, they are conditional. Thus, certain conditions must be sufficiently effective before stuttering can be produced.

    Bluemel further defined stuttering as: 'evidence of the child's speech or thought block, occurring when verbal imagery or mental speech recoils from the stream of consciousness; thus, breaking continuity'. He maintained that, 'Stuttering is the child attempting to speak without the "mental imagery'" which makes speech possible'.

12. Stuttering behaviors: defined in terms of anticipatory struggle reactions, which even in their simplest symptoms are indications of the child's efforts to avoid stuttering (Bloodstein, 1975).

    Bloodstein contended that the child's negative perceptions of his dysfluencies led to attempts to avoid or struggle through the anticipated dysfluencies. These attempts constituted both the child's adjustments, i.e. speech-related struggles, and his stuttering behaviors.

    Bloodstein's emphasis on the child's anticipatory struggle reactions provided very significant insights into the formation and activation of stuttering behaviors. He regarded such reactions as an integral part of the stuttering behaviors. He showed that, even at an early age, the child was neither passively, nor involuntarily, subjugated to his stuttering behaviors, as was commonly believed. Those viewed are regarded to be compatible with the application of neuropsychology to the study of stuttering.

13. Stuttering was defined, by Weiss (1964), as a form of 'dissociate aphasia' – a term used in his comparison of cluttering with stuttering. He stated: 'I believe there is a disturbance of the thought processes; the deficiency is word-finding and sentence formation, and later on, an interference between the thoughts which the patient wants to utter, and ideas of existing speech difficulties' (Froeschels, 1964).

14. Stuttering is commonly associated with abnormal breathing in the tonic block, and coupled with facial grimaces and clenched fists, whereas the clonic movements are repetitive. These basic stuttering behaviors are also designed to help stutterers draw attention away from their stuttering behaviors (Froeschels, 1964).

15. Stuttering is a cramp-like (spasmatic), expressive neurosis within

the area of oral communication, stemming from a nervous reaction within a constitutional basis (Luchsinger and Arnold, 1965).

16. Stuttering symptoms and associative behaviors constitute conditioned emotional responses evoked by classical neurophysiological conditioning (Brutten and Shoemaker, 1967).

    This definition centered its emphasis predominantly on the early stages of the neurophysiological formation of stuttering behaviors. There appears to be valid reasons for considering these stages to be more indicative of pre-stuttering, rather than the actual advent of developmental stuttering. (This is discussed in later sections.)

17. Stuttering: 'A disruption in the fluency of verbal expressions; characterized by involuntary audible or silent, syllabic, or word repetitions and prolongations, commonly accompanied by related and unrelated, facial and bodily movements' (Wingate, 1964). Wingate also formulated a working definition for stuttering (see next section).
18. Stuttering behaviors: 'Disruptions to the stutterer's normal fluent speech, which are evident as speech-related struggles' (Shames and Rubin,1986). Although not a new approach, the authors emphasized the positive aspects of the stutterer, and provided behavioral insights into stuttering not commonly presented within most past and current definitions of stuttering.

In summary there is obvious overlapping between some of the above definitions. Some appear to refer to the same things in different ways, whereas others are overtly different. Considering the vast differences between many of these definitions, the reader might wonder, 'Can all these definitions be referring to a singular behavioral disorder, namely, stuttering?'.

Comments: years of working with stutterers have lead to the contention that traumatic experiences related to negative speech-gratification experiences can vary in form and degree, and often relate to the severity and sustainment of stuttering behaviors. Experiences that may be traumatic to one individual, however, might not incur traumatic consequences for another. How can we determine which traumatic experiences may or may not lead to stuttering, or to some other forms of behavioral disorders?

The diversity of reported symptoms and behavioral deficits reported for stuttering has presented as much of a puzzle as its cause(s). Understanding stuttering, however, pertains to more than excessive attention to its obvious symptoms and behavioral deficits. There are also apparently less obvious neuropsychological factors: volition, motivation, preoccupation, anticipation, socioenvironmental experiences, emotional states, traumatic reactions, etc. These factors may be of greater importance, particularly for obtaining beneficial and consistent therapy results (see the following chapters).

Van Riper and Wingate: working definitions for stuttering

Aware of the many different and often contradictory criteria for evaluating and remediating stuttering behaviors, Van Riper and Wingate formulated working definitions intended to provide standard formats for the diagnosis of the symptoms of stuttering

Van Riper: overt stuttering symptomatologies

Van Riper's (1973) overt stuttering symptomatologies were a concerted effort to formulate a diagnostic inventory for categorizing a range of discrete stuttering symptoms, and associated behaviors, as listed below:

- Tremors
  Localized areas of tension
  Postural fixation
  Pressure surge (air or muscle tension)
- Blockages and closures: momentary (or long) occlusion of airway
- Interrupter devices: movements designed to terminate a block
- Postural fixation: partial constriction of airway (primarily seen in continuants); tremors are often observed here
- Vocal fry: used to initiate voice sounds between tension surges on blocks
- Repetitive stuttering: pulses of air before unvoiced consonants
- Complemental air: used to initiate speech-forced-out-word on last of breath; usually on continuants
- Trigger postures: inappropriate articulatory posture to initiate speech; usually precede tremors
- Recoil behavior: seen at start of tremor; immediate attempt to reentry to sound tension surges and irregularity in the occurrence observed
- Disguised reactions: behaviors used to cover appearances of stuttering; physical movements or attitude shifts preceding or simultaneous with stuttering
- Avoidance behaviors: constituted behaviors such as:
  Refusal behaviors; substitutions, circumlocution
  Postponement devices: (uh),(well), (yoy know), (let me see), with physical movements indicating more speech wil be forthcoming
- Timing devices and 'starters': behavior synchronized with postponement devices to get into speech–physical movements or speech (similar to interruptors)
- Abulia: severe silent postures; seeming loss of awareness.

Van Riper regarded disturbing external influences, by parents and others, to be a primary factor in the transition of children's normal non-fluencies (primary stuttering) to secondary (classical) stuttering symptoms. This related well to his preventive programs with young children, He tended, however, within his diagnostic and therapy approaches with adult stutterers to be more attentive to the neurophysiological components of stuttering behaviors. Yet, the more rigid and complex nature of the adults' stuttering behaviors generally appeared stubbornly resistant to such techniques as relaxation and desensitization, which centered on adaptation methods to reduce, control or suppress the individual's stuttering behaviors,

In summary Van Riper's overt stuttering symptomatologies served towards giving better characterization and diagnosis of the physiology of stuttering behaviors. His working definition regarding its practical remedial applications with older teenagers and adult stutterers seemed, however, to be limited because of its close adherence to a neurophysiological format for stuttering behaviors.

Wingate's working definition for stuttering

Wingate's working definition for stuttering was as empirical as Van Riper's was discrete. His working definition regards stuttering as:

> Disruption in the fluency of verbal expression, which is characterized by involuntary, audible or silent repetitions or prolongations in the utterance of short speech elements; namely, sounds syllables, and words of one syllable.
>
> These disruptions usually occur frequently and are not readily controllable.
>
> Sometimes the disruptions are accompanied by accessory activities involving the speech apparatus, related or unrelated bodily structures, or stereotyped speech utterances. These give the appearances of being speech-related struggles.
>
> Also, there are frequently indications or reports of the presence of an emotional state ranging from a general condition of excitement to more specific emotions of a negative nature, such as fear, embarrassment, irritation or the like.
>
> The immediate source of stuttering is some incoordination expressed in the peripheral mechanism; the ultimate cause is presently unknown and may be complex or compound.
>
> *Wingate (1964)*

Comments: Wingate's working definition gained general support primarily within the USA. As a working definition, it tends to refer, more or less, to the obvious involuntary classical stuttering symptoms, and thus, tends to lean towards a mainly neurophysiological perspective for stuttering behaviors. This definition, therefore, would tend to be consistent with the currect use of mechanistic/manipulative techniques for treating stuttering behaviors.

Primary non-fluencies and classical stuttering symptoms

Van Riper characterized primary non-fluencies as a stage in the child's progressive development of speech. He related this stage to a normal maturational lag between the children's developing neurophysiological components for expressive speech and his communicative efforts to cope with expanding environmental experiences. Primary non-fluencies tend to show basic behavioral similarities with classical stuttering symptoms, and thus may be mistaken for them.

Classical stuttering symptoms are generally regarded as evidence of the formation of involuntary stuttering behaviors. Van Riper termed these symptoms 'secondary stuttering'. Wingate, as noted above, characterized the classical stuttering symptoms as:

> Disruptions in the fluency of verbal expressions which are characterized as involuntary, audible or silent, repetitions or prolongations in the utterances of short speech elements, namely; sounds, syllables, and words of one syllable. These disruptions usually occur frequently and are not readily controllable.

Although primary non-fluencies may appear to exhibit neurophysiological behavioral similarities, they are not subject to similar neuropsychological factors, as noted below

- Primary non-fluencies are indicative of a normal stage within the children's maturational time-table for the progressive development of their speech skills.
- Classical stuttering symptoms relate to conflicting involuntary neurophysiological non-motor speech processes, which disrupt the children's performances of their normally developing or developed fluent speech.
- Children exhibiting classical stuttering symptoms usually have become aware and reactive to their stuttering behaviors, which evoke confused behaviors and related emotional states, whereas, children exhibiting primary non-fluencies generally do not.
- Classical stuttering symptoms become more evident as episodes of tonic and/or clonic oral blockages, with associated bodily tensions. Primary non-fluencies usually show little, if any, bodily tensions, and tend to dissipate into stable fluent speech.
- Classical stuttering symptoms can lead to progressive negative emotions, attitudes, preoccupations, anticipations, disturbed readiness SETs* for speech, etc. Stuttering behaviors have been attributed to

*SETs are defined by Goldstein (1948) as his concept that 'each performance is due to the function of the total organism in which the brain plays a particular role'. To perform a particular function, therefore, the individual must act volitionally as with the runner or as a function of the action as perceptually perceived and intended. Although all functions may not be overtly evident, they nevertheless contribute 'supportive' functions.

many causes: heredity, mental illnesses, mental handicap, traumatic experiences, neurological deficits, neuroses, disturbed learning, etc. Primary non-fluencies are more commonly indicative of normal maturational lag.

- Attempt is usually made to treat classical stuttering symptoms clinically, but I strongly advise against calling undue attention to primary non-fluency behaviors.

Neurophysiological and neuropsychological bases for normal fluency and potential dysfluency behaviors

Programs for treating stuttering would be expected to show greater considerations not only towards certain negative factors, which tend to precipitate episodes of stuttering behaviors, but also to positive factors that promote fluent-speech performances. The more dominant of these are discussed below.

Speech-gratification dependence: a natural human inclination and primary motivational power

> Nothing serves to promote selective action or responses, as does successful attainment of one's appetites.
>
> *Trumble and Noble (1966)*

Gratification

This is the positive effect of satisfying/rewarding experiences. During the pre-speech stage, young children lack the cognitive abilities to differentiate their use of object-words to express themselves. What the children perceive, seek and experience as gratifying relates to a natural inclination, which, at their young age, Piaget (1948) referred to as a primary motivational power.

What motivates the young infant, an extremely dependent creature, who during his early developmental years develops a basic skill as complex as speech? As a newly born, however, the young child was not entirely unprepared to leave the comforts of the mother's womb. He left with a remarkable fund of genetically specified basic skills which, with proper stimulations and nurturing, within relatively definable chronological periods, attain their potential mature developments.

The newborn does not enter the world sermonizing on, 'The blessings of birth', and yet, during his earliest formative years, expends extensive activity in language–speech acquisition (Strang, 1959). This early onset of conscious awareness of oral–language relationships was attributed by Rosenthal (1977) to the expanding and stimulating influences of the child's environmental milieu, within which he seeks gratification experiences through speech from his increasing human contacts. This concept is supported by others, such as Kessen (1963), who stated:

> Evidence of the existence of self-initiated goal-striving behavior in the infant has replaced the outmoded view of baby as a creature who waits passively to have his bodily needs cared for by others.

Speech skills, in spite of being genetically specified, do not develop instinctively. Nor are young children prone to continue their prespeech vocalizations – babbling, echolalia and jargon – without sustained reinforcing experiences. In this regard, Rosenthal (1977) stated:

> The children's echolalic and babbling behaviors require little, if any, conscious thought with regard to their application as a functional, let alone a social tool.
>
> These early egocentric vocalizations characterize the children's genetic specificity for speech, as well as provide the perceptual–motor movements for preparing the neurophysiologic bases for speech development.

Aristotle regarded humans as having a natural inclination to seek, for themselves, that which they perceive to be good, i.e. gratifying. Speech, by virtue of its natural accessibility as a medium for communicating, becomes the most readily available means by which children seek gratification of their basic needs. Their dependence on gratification experiences serves to motivate and reinforce sustainment of their dependence on speech and, thus, is a potent neuropsychological factor which can effectively influence the neurophysiological processes for the development of speech and its performances.

Young children are highly egocentric in their craving for gratification of their basic needs (comforts, sense of well-being, sentient pleasures, affection, etc.). They are, however, primarily dependent on external sources for these gratifications, which they learn are generally accorded in response to their early vocalizations. Parents, and others, promote the children's early dependence on speech by properly stimulating and gratifying their speech efforts. Children thus learn to use speech as a primary means for communicating to gratify needs and desires. Without early and consistent gratification experiences, the progression of the children's developing speech skills can be severely compromised.

Comments: consciously or not, as we mature throughout our lives, the gratification we derive from our use of speech continues to serve as a primary motivational power. This is no less so for stutterers who, unlike non-stutterers, expend considerable preoccupation and efforts striving to reassert their natural inclination for gratification of their needs and aspirations through the readily accessible use of speech.

External influences on the use and development of speech

> The healthy child is active and curious and seeks stimulation from the environment.

The progressive development of children's speech, according to the Lurias, requires complementary neurophysiological interplay between genetic and environmental influences. The genetic influences are most effective during the earlier stages of their pre-speech vocalizations. During the later stages, in their use and development of speech skills, external stimuli will be most effective.

We can observe the cultural influences of external stimuli, for example, in the reduction of almost 88 sound phonemes evident in young children's early babbling, echolalic and jargon vocalizations. This reduction is the result of exposure to the lower number of sound phonemes used within the language common to their particular societies and occurs without the children's conscious selection. Their imitative reproductions are limited to their perceptions (modes of perception) of those sound phonemes common to their societies. Culturally specific languages – English, Norwegian, Chinese, etc. – are products of external influences, and do not relate to genetic specificity.

External influences similarly determine, motivate, expand and diversify the children's interests, as well as their needs. These influences greatly enhance vocabulary growth, and increase use of multisyllabic words and complex sentences. Additionally, these influences promote differentiation in language usage (intellect), and syntactic constructions in their speech performances.

Before exhibiting normal primary non-fluency, most children have experienced relative freedom from negative external pressures, which might have been imposed upon, or related to, their speech efforts. Between their third and fifth years, therefore, they generally have developed sufficient assertive expressive speech to complement and closely relate to external influences. The extent to which they do so provides them with, as Rosenthal contends and Seligman (1975) supports, an adaptive assertive control within their environments.

Children's continued dependence on speech-gratification experiences therefore relates to their perceptions and adjustments to expanding socioenvironments. Rogers (1947) referred to their psychological dependence on external influences in their use of basic speech skills as goal-directed attempts to satisfy needs as experienced within their perceptions of the environment. The child's speech performances are usually consistent with his concept of self and ways of behavior, which at his young age are highly egocentric. When these are inconsistent, he tends to have difficulty with perceptions and reactions to external speech stimuli. Rogers concluded:

Most of the ways of behaving which are adopted by the organism are those which are consistent with the concept of self.

Heightened-speech behaviors: a behavioral consequence of maturational limitations

The young child is verbal, highly active, enjoys solving problems, though he is unable to verbalize his solutions. *Elkind (1967)*

The on-going development of the young child is commonly a source of parental amazement and joy. His earliest efforts to walk, to take his first awkward steps towards them into his future delights them, as does his dependence on them for intimate support. Parents usually show little concern when their child displays obvious awkwardness in his early efforts to walk. When the child, however, at a later but still tender age, shows comparable awkwardness in the performances of his developing speech, usually as primary non-fluences, the parents may respond with unwarranted, though well-meaning, concerns and attentions.

Young children are generally not aware of their developing speech, which they are motivated to use primarily through its association with gratification experiences. The developmental status of their speech tends to progress at a chronological level generally sufficient for gratifying their on-going maturational needs. They therefore have no need to become consciously preoccupied or concerned with the correct articulatory or grammatical aspects of their developing speech performances.

Long before children exhibit primary non-fluencies, their dependence on speech-gratification experiences, as an effective neuropsychological factor, has become basic to their homeostasis, which Goldstein (1948) defined as: 'The consistent striving of organisms to come to terms with themselves, and their environments.'

The proper interplay between the child's perceptual responses to external stimuli and the neurophysiological motor processes for his speech performances is conducive to normally developing speech. When subject to disturbed perceptions and emotional responses, caused by confusing external stimuli, this interplay may be disrupted. External influences, causing the child to become unsure of his speech, can lead to confusion and threaten his speech-gratification dependence. The child will attempt to cope by centering his efforts on his speech, for which he had little prior experience. In this regard, Goldstein (1939) commented:

There are indications of the early efforts of young children to conform to socio-environmental influences.

When the child is subjected to disturbing speech or related experiences, his maturational limitations to cope properly with these threats to his homeostasis tend to become negatively obvious. As a result of these limitations, and lacking prior experiences to effect conforming changes in his speech, the child is restricted to the current status of his development. The consequence of this is often noted in the child heightening the manner of his current speech. This tends to reflect his striving for approval (gratification) from his speech efforts. The general characteristics of his heightened speech are restated below:

1. Noticeable increase in speech rate.
2. The tendency to run out of speech breath, or attempts to speak with insufficient speech breath.
3. A seeming urgency in his speech performance, but no overt increase in the intensity of his primary non-fluency behaviors: repetitions, hesitations, prolongations, mild blockings, etc.
4. May seem to use starters. These, however, tend to indicate more confused spontaneous reponses and seeking of means, rather than conscious coping adjustment efforts.

Comments: heightened speech behaviors have tended to be mistaken for signs of dysfluency and even chronic stuttering. This is unfortunate because the child may have to endure current and later negative neuropsychological consequences which can lead to the disturbed neurophysiological motor processes related to behavioral disorders such as stuttering. Shames and Rubin's (1986) comment related to this topic is also worth repeating:

> The point is that not all behaviors that affect the forward flow of speech are indicative of disorganization or disorder. Even the presence of dysfluencies that are indicative of break-down are not necessarily evidence of a disorder. They may merely be the result of a momentary and sporadic lack of the organization that fluency production requires.

Maturational status of children exhibiting heightened speech behaviors

Limited research attention has apparently been given to the maturational status of children within the time frames in which they may exhibit heightened speech behaviors, because only vague references relating to the topic could be found. These seemingly disorganized speech behaviors should, however, be viewed, as Shames and Rubin alluded, within the context of the children's current mental, neurophysiological and social maturational states.

Young children, active and curious, seek stimulation from their environments. Their world is a giant Pandora's Box full of wondrous, surprising adventures to be experienced. They lift the lid to peek and poke about within, eager to touch upon experiences they cannot fully comprehend, let alone clearly verbalize. These limitations, however, reflect their immaturities, rather than any particular or generalized neural or functional disturbances.

Rosenthal contended, however, that children have a strong need to assert themselves through speech. Their speech efforts, when limited by normal immaturities and improperly imposed upon, may lead to heightened speech, which can become a minefield of potential frustrations and negative emotional states, leading to evoked traumatic neuropsychological consequences, such as stuttering.

Speech is a deceptively complex skill, which children appear to develop with little conscious effort. Its development, however, requires harmonious interactions between their multiple bodily, sensory and neurological systems. Although each system matures within its own biological time frame, they depend greatly upon each other for the fulfilment of their potential functional performances, as well as developments.

> All aspects of physical, psychological, and social development are so interrelated and dependent upon each other that discussing each one in turn is highly artificial and perhaps even misleading.
>
> *Buhler (1968)*

Primary non-fluencies do not result from maturational deficits. Rather, they reflect a normal developmental stage within which the child's various bodily systems are striving to function uniformly to perform the neurophysiological motor speech processes. Also, during this stage, children's receptive language is overtly in advance of their expressive speech modalities. Consequently, the child's limited ability to express himself can lead to his heightened speech behaviors which, if unchecked, may relate to the neuropsychological conditions that lead to more overt dysfluency behaviors.

As children progress in maturity, they show increasing volitional use of speech, which serves towards reinforcing their functional dependence on speech. They thus show increased:

- Self-assertiveness in their use of speech and a sense of control of their environment.
- Self-visualization with regard to perceiving and attending, visually, auditorally and proprioceptively to the motor movements of their speech efforts.
- Cognition perceptions of particular objects, words and related events, within expanding environments.
- Volitional differentiation: discrimination processes among object-words, symbols and internal programs of action.

- Ideation: (to assume the possible) planning the means deemed necessary for obtaining the desired objectives by the use of speech.
- Attention to the qualitative aspects of speech, such as sentence structures and syntactic forms.

In summary: disturbing external influences imposed upon the child's speech or related efforts may, as a result of maturational limitations, cause the child to effect heightened speech behaviors, which tend to manifest maturational non-fluencies, rather than dysfluencies. Proper diagnostic attention is required to prevent erroneous assessments of such speech behaviors, and the potential negative consequences, which may result from unnecessary and inappropriate remedial methods.

Relationships between negative emotional states and stuttering behaviors

The notion that negative external stimuli and emotional states are key factors in the traumatic onset and formation of stuttering behaviors is not a newly conceived idea. References to such factors appear in some early theoretical approaches to stuttering. These factors are currently being given increased consideration regarding their neuropsychological relationships to various aspects of stuttering behaviors.

In spite of extensive research, there is a lack of clinical evidence to support such long-held notions that stuttering is primarily the result of inherent, or pathological, deficits. Gerhardt, Van Riper and Johnson, among others, contend that most children exhibiting chronic stuttering behaviors are free of prior inherent, congenital or post-birth anomalies that might account for these behaviors.

Whether or not negative external stimuli or emotional states imposed upon the child are overtly evident, their potential traumatic influences must always be suspect. Who can say what constitutes a traumatizing speech-related experience that is sufficient to precipitate the onset and/or repeated episodes of chronic stuttering behaviors?

Wingate's working definition for classical stuttering symptoms refers to negative emotional states, but does not clearly relate them to possible traumatic etiological factors. In this regard, as noted earlier, he stated:

> . . . there are frequent indications or reports of the presence of an emotional state ranging from a general condition of excitement to more specific emotions of a negative nature, i.e. fear, embarrassment, irritation, or the like.
>
> The immediate source of stuttering is some incoordinations expressed in the peripheral mechanisms: the ultimate cause is presently unknown and may be complex or compound.

Comments: Wingate's (1964) somewhat tentative reference to external factors and negative emotional states tends to denote primarily a neurophysiological basis for stuttering, as does Van Riper's. Van Riper, however, more specifically related negative emotional states to inappropriate parental attentions towards the child's speech efforts (i.e. non-fluencies). Consistent with neuropsychological concepts, some forms of traumatic experiences and associated negative emotional states are major factors in the onset, and repeated episodes, of stuttering behaviors.

Traumatic neuropsychological reactions to feelings of helplessness and related negative emotional states

Seligman (1975) closely associated feelings of helplessness with the loss of the predictability of controlling one's environment. A primary function of predictability is the ability to perceive cognitively and anticipate the possible outcome of one's participation within different milieu. There is a definite traumatic basis for feelings of helplessness.

For successful perception and anticipation, i.e. prediction, of the outcome of one's speech performances within different environmental situations, specific cognition of reality and internal programs of action is required. Without these essential experiences the child or adult stutterer, lacking predictability with regard to his speech efforts, tends to be more readily subject to the frustrating intimidations of demands on his speech.

The child or adult stutterer, lacking alternative internal programs of action, cannot act properly to conform his speech behaviors as needed. Without prior differential speech experiences, he has only the current status of his speech upon which to model changes in his speech behaviors. This restriction compounds his feelings of helplessness, confusion and related negative emotional states, when anticipating, as well as within speech events.

In summary, stuttering behaviors, in view of the above, are seen as traumatic neuropsychological reactions to external intimidating influences on speech or speech-related experiences. Negative emotional states will, therefore, always be indicated, whether or not they are overtly evident. Intimidating experiences manifest themselves as helplessness and related negative emotional states, which can evoke traumatizing reactions at any age.

Acting with volition, preoccupation and change in motivational emphasis for speech

A common reference to stuttering behaviors relates to their involuntary occurrences. This basic characteristic of stuttering behaviors is, however, the product of disturbances of particular functions and events, including the individual's volitional efforts to act.

One theory on stuttering alludes that stutterers may have chosen to stutter as a less stressful alternative to coming to terms with some unmanageable situation or persistent problem. This is subject to doubt because, from its early onset, it is quite apparent from the characteristics of their volitional coping methods that stutterers generally choose not to stutter.

It might, however, seem contradictory, if not absurd, to contend that preoccupation with not stuttering may constitute a major contributing factor not only to the progressive formation of stuttering behaviors, but also to the repeated occurrences of their involuntary episodes.

The child's heightened speech behaviors are seen as a volitional change from his earlier, relatively uninhibited, inherent dependence on speech for gratifying basic needs, without any need to attend consciously to the manner of his performance.

Heightened speech is, thus, indicative of the child's immature preoccupations with his speech performance, as he attempts volitionally to cope with the confusing external influences being directed at his speech. The child is endeavoring to experience gratification in the form of relief from perceived rejection of his speech efforts, rather than from a natural inclination to gratify basic needs.

The young child has little cognitive awareness of his limited speech, which develops relative to his needs and experiences. Such awareness, the Lurias contended, requires the crucial power of recognizing reality, which he had not developed sufficiently at this stage because of maturational limitations,

In summary the child, who is compelled by external demands to attend prematurely to his speech, will tend to exhibit more intensive heightened speech behaviors, which may lead to increased confusion and related negative emotional states. His confused preoccupation may elicit ambiguous motor–sensory excitations, which can conflict with the formation of his relatively automated neurophysiological formed motor processes for his developing fluent speech.

The child's loss of self-assertiveness, and visualization of the success of his speech efforts, may be disturbed most. Other aspects of his developed neurophysiological motor processes for fluent speech generally remain intact, although subject to disruptive episodes.

Comments: the child, at this stage, should not be regarded or treated as a stutterer, because his basic speech behaviors are still very responsive to correct stimulating influences. As Van Riper strongly advised, at this stage, the more productive therapy is administered to the child's parents and/or others involved.

Coping adjustment methods

> All behavior can be said to involve deciding what to do and then doing it.
>
> *Trumble and Noble (1966)*

Allport's theory of behavior tends to relate to the negative consequences of coping adjustment methods to control and/or avoid stuttering behaviors. He stated:

> Behaviors once acquired to serve another purpose become an end in themselves and act as motives.

The stutterer's preoccupations with confusing and/or disturbing attentions towards his speech efforts are evident through their volitional use of coping adjustment methods. By such methods, the stutterer strives to control or suppress his stuttering behavior, and/or avoid negative consequences imposed upon his speech efforts.

Volitional coping adjustment methods tend, however, to become involuntary stuttering behaviors with repetition. This change is caused by the persistence of stutterers to continue using such methods in spite of their frequent tendency to diminish in value as speech aids, particularly as starters. Such methods tend to lose their initial values to effect fluent speech because they constitute non-speech artifacts, rather than basic neurophysiological motor speech functions.

As the stutterer persists in using diminishing coping adjustment methods to effect fluent speech, his continued efforts tend to become speech-related struggles, which are more pronounced as involuntary, non-speech, neurophysiological, motor (facial and body) movements. These struggles may then perseverate as added associated stuttering behaviors within his repertoire of stuttering behaviors.

> *Comments*: we should note that preoccupation with use of volitional methods to avoid stuttering is an untenable objective desire from which the stutterer is seeking gratification. This tends to produce restrictive results, because it is contrary to the natural inclination for speech as an available medium for communicating and gratifying the stutterer's needs and desires.

The cumulative psychosocial aspects of developmental stuttering

There is considerably more to stuttering than its overt, involuntary, audible and visual, classical symptoms. Stuttering, as discussed earlier, does not constitute a form of speech disorder per se. Stutterers do exhibit normal fluent speech, but as a result of disturbed neuropsychological processes they are hindered from doing so within speech situations.

As noted earlier, there are no proven inherent or organic neuropathic disorders that might account for the vast majority of stutterers or explain why they do not stutter within all potentially traumatic speech situations. It is rather apparent that to stutter requires a social interaction between a minimum of two people. What then is the nature of these social factors which, within particular speech situations, disrupt an individual's normally developed fluent speech?

We are, therefore, left to consider that developmental stuttering, although manifesting neurophysiological dysfluent speech, is more realistically a form of psychosocial behavioral disorder, primarily related to the individual's traumatic speech-related psychosocial experiences.

Children are not likely to develop disturbed psychosocial attitudes solely because of their stuttering behaviors. The formation of disturbed psychosocial attitudes and related negative behaviors relate more directly to how they are regarded, react and treated within their socioenvironments.

Stutterers may start to incur negative attitudes and behaviors during their early developmental years, as a result of being treated as awkward children. The psychosocial effects of these negative experiences can influence their attitudes and emotional states from childhood to adulthood. In this regard, Strang (1959) stated:

> The awkward child may be rejected by other children, which thus, tends to negatively affect his social development.

Rosenthal emphasized the early need for assertiveness in children's use of speech, particularly as a social medium. Children showing stuttering behaviors tend to be less secure in their dependence on speech for obtaining gratifications of their needs. They may show reduced speech assertiveness and self-confidence, lower self-esteem, etc., and depict, as alluded to by Strang, the awkward child.

As these children mature towards adulthood, personal, social, academic and vocational standards place increasing demands on their speech skills. Difficulty to meet these demands tend, not only to restrict their potentials to meet these needs and aspirations, but also to lead to misconceptions regarding their lack of intelligence, talents and initiative, and thus to be disadvantaged throughout their lives.

Stutterers have been disadvantaged by well-meaning misconceptions. Such notions contend that stutterers should realistically limit their needs, social and vocational aspirations to objectives requiring minimum speech skills to ensure reasonable success with minimum frustration. When stutterers are subjected to the effects of these notions, what kind of psychosocial attitudes and emotional adjustments can be expected of them?

Through such notions, stutterers are often counselled to make compromising adjustments, which actually require their acceptance of being disadvantaged. Their psychosocial responses to lost opportunities may tend to be reflected in forms of submissiveness: complacency, compliance, sublimation or restrained forms of passive aggressions; and evidence of compensating and/or withdrawal avoidance behaviors. Such compromising adjustments are, however, certainly not indicative of the considerably more positive self-image stutterers hold, but are constrained to suppress.

These compromising behaviors are generally fostered from early childhood into the teenage years. Within classrooms, play and other group activities, they may feign inattentiveness, lack of preparation, illness, indifference, etc., or disturbing behaviors, to avoid adverse consequences of exhibiting stuttering behaviors. They are prone to linger at the outer fringes of these social environments, eager to enter and participate, but intimidated from doing so. They might tend to confuse rejection of their speech behaviors with rejection of themselves.

The above does not infer any contrived societal design to disadvantage stutterers. Rather, societal notions of what is realistic for stutterers are, as noted, often well-meaning and thus difficult for them to cope with, particularly during the teenage years, when the negative implications of stuttering become increasingly more apparent.

Feelings of helplessness, as Seligman (1975) contended, reflect confusion and loss of predictability to control different environments. This can be evident in stutterers when adjusting to cope with different speech situations. Consequently, they becomes less secure in anticipating the outcome of their participation in certain speech situations.

Increased feelings of helplessness, and related negative emotional responses to compromising experiences, effect changes in the neuropsychological parameters of the stutterer's anticipations regarding perception, and outcome, of participation in speech events. These perceptions therefore become more rigidly influenced by negative anticipations which contribute greatly to repeated episodes of stuttering behaviors.

All humans show individual differences, whether or not they may have certain genetic, organic or functional characteristics in common. Consequently, there is no singular personality profile common to either stutterers or non-stutterers. Stutterers, as noted above, might, however, display certain general psychological attitudes and behavioral characteristics that may be attributable to psychosocial problems in adjusting to their experiences as stutterers.

Tom Green, Special Psychologist at a center in Norway (Halmrast Senter for Stammebehandling) reported in his pre-doctoral study indications for certain common psychological attitudes and behaviors in tests with young and adult stutterers. These findings, presented at the

International Conference on Stuttering, Paris, in September 1991, suggest certain general personality and behavioral patterns among the subjects studied. The abstract of this paper stated:

> A complete account of the cumulative effect of being a stutterer has also taken into consideration how the person influences his stuttering.
>
> 26 severe stutterers at Halmrast Center for treating stuttering, went through the battery of P.W.S.P.I. (vs 1.0.) tests. Results showed a significant interaction between personality actors and self-evaluated stuttering related behaviors.
>
> This is promising regarding the possibility of empirically establishing relationships between the effects of being a stutterer and the general adaptation of the person to social demands.

In summary, the close relationships between psychosocial factors and stuttering behaviors should no longer be subject to doubt. Psychosocial experiences, whether positive or negative, can influence specific forms of human behaviors, rather than evoking indifferent neuropsychological reactions.

Comments: the seemingly compulsive search for causes and symptoms of stuttering has long overshadowed the need to account properly for the psychosocial influences that tend to shape the lives of stutterers. More attention should be given to the disturbing psychosocial attitudes and behaviors, which may lead them towards compromising adjustments and suppression of their aspirations during their school years and throughout adulthood.

Examples of the effects of disturbing perceptions of external stimuli on non-speech motor performances

To better understand another, one should walk a mile in his moccasins.

Old Indian Adage

We are not usually too eager to try and put ourselves in the shoes of another with an unmanageable disorder in an attempt to understand him or his affliction better. We would be more prudent to compare his affliction with certain other closely related, and better understood, disorders.

We might also have better understanding of disturbances to the motor performances of one skill through comparison with the disturbed motor performance of a closely related skill. Walking, likened to speech, is a perceptual–motor skill. Although not as complex as speech, walking does relate comparatively to the formation of the basic neurophysiological perceptual–motor processes relative to each skill. Both are basic skills, which in the absence of chronic debilitating problems are commonly taken for granted. Walking may therefore be used to illustrate temporary neurophysiological breakdowns of its otherwise normal functions and can provide insights into the potentials of external stimuli to effectively disturb the neurophysiological motor processes for a developed skill, such as speech.

Rummaging through the trivia of our past, we may recall having experienced, at one time or another, brief discomforting disruptions to our normally developed walking skills. We might, for example, recall the experience of walking down a strange street, and suddenly feeling acutely aware of suspicious eyes watching our passage, to which we might have reacted as follows:

> We might become very self-conscious, sensing ourselves to be exposed, uncomfortably out of place, and experience a sense of overt awkwardness in our walking movements. We find that despite conscious efforts our movements continue to be somewhat sluggish and incoordinated in a manner that might be described as non-fluent. When, however, feeling free of the watchful eyes, normal walking movements tend to return.

Readers might also have had similar or related experiences. Many years ago, visiting a dance hall, I chose to favor a fetching beauty seated across the dance floor with the privilege of a dance. After venturing confidently to her table, my offer was flatly declined. I recall my reactions as follows:

> Experiencing disappointment, with my ego a bit out of joint, I turned to return to my table. I suddenly perceived all eyes had witnessed my being rejected.
>
> With strained efforts to display an aura of cool indifference, I sought the sanctuary of my table across the room. As I began to walk my steps seemed to become uncertain, rubbery, as if my normally developed walking skill had become somewhat palsied; I was experiencing perceptual–motor incoordinations.
>
> My awkward walking continued despite my volitional efforts to walk with more certain steps. The distance to my table seemed to have increased geometrically in proportion to the discomfort to my wounded ego.

We might also refer to the worker whose skilled hands suddenly become all thumbs when he perceives the boss critically observing his work. Negative preoccupations with perceptions of the close proximity of the boss can evoke awkward perceptual–motor responses, which can temporarily disrupt the relatively automated performance of the worker's developed skills.

Perhaps the readers might recall other comparative experiences. Developed performances of a skill, be it walking, precision work or speech, depends on their basic perceptual–motor movements, being formed as relatively automated neurophysiological processes in basic motor programs. The relative automation of these basic perceptual–motor processes enables the individual:

- To perform the particular skill with little need to consciously attend to each of its movements, but rather to attend primarily upon cognition of the objectives for performing the skill.
- To maintain a stable pre-SET status of readiness to perform the intended actions of the skill.

Within each of the above examples, the individual's responses to his disturbing perceptions of the external stimuli briefly disrupted his performances of a developed non-speech motor skill. Hebb (1949) maintained that changing the performances of a particular skill cannot occur without the person having attained some degree of its functional development. Where there is no development, disruptive changes in the performances of the skill cannot obviously occur.

Learning more commonly implies conscious efforts to pursue and add to what is being or has been learned. Genetically specific basic skills, such as walking and speech in their early development, form primarily as a function of usage based on inherent drives to gratify needs, and thus require minimal conscious efforts. This serves towards automating the skill's basic neurophysiological functions, which enables the child to be concerned with the where to and why his feet are taking him, rather than being preoccupied with how they must function to get him there.

Individuals' disturbing perceptions may be based on real or imagined external stimuli. Their affects upon the developed neurophysiological perceptual–motor performances for the particular skill may nevertheless be disruptive. As long as the disturbing perceptions persist, the individual will experience resistance controling the awkward motor functions relative to the disturbed skill.

These events that disturb neuropsychological experiences are usually of short duration. As the child regains control of his perceptions, the neurophysiological motor processes for the skill return to their relatively automated performance. This relates to the earlier reference to Gerhardt's rigidity of neural cells.

Can we apply the above brief perceptual–motor disruptions, which are related to disturbing perceptions and responses to external stimuli, in a similar way to otherwise normally developed speech? In this regard, the comments of Shame and Rubins (1986) are deemed worth restating:

> . . . it is the two-factor position that motor speech performance is fundamentally like all other motor performances; its efficiency is interfered with by the presence of excessive emotions.
>
> The point is that not all behaviors that affect the forward flow of speech is indicative of disorganization or disorder. Even the presence of dysfluencies that are indicative of breakdown are not necessarily evidence of a disorder. They may merely be the result of a momentary and sporadic lack of the organization that fluency production requires.

In the above and in preceding sections, I have touched on certain neuropsychological and neurophysiological events to provide rational insights for understanding the bases for chronic repetition of stuttering behaviors, which I deem to be essential for administering benefical and consistant therapy programs. Although these topics are discussed in greater detail in later sections, it is hoped the readers will find such repetition helpful, rather than unduly distracting.

Comments: comparable experiences by the readers of awkward behavioral reactions to disturbing perceptions of external stimulli can help towards better understanding of the dual-tract motor program approach for speech and developmental stuttering.

Chapter 4
The neurophysiological basis of developmental stuttering

Some years ago, I came across a quotation, which seemed appropriate to present, with an added thought, to provide a helpful insight to a class about stuttering. Regrettably, the name of the author of the original quotation, deserving of due credit, now eludes me. His or her quotation was:

> If movements do not get into the children's muscles, they cannot get into their brains.

To this I added:

> When bad movements get into the muscles, they may have gotten into the brain as stuttering behaviors.

Within the preceding chapter, we discussed neurophysiological disruptions to the individual's motor performances, i.e. walking, precipitated by disturbing perceptions of external stimuli.

> Might the individual's awkward walking develop into chronic episodes of dysfluent-walking behaviors, if similarly subjected to repeated and prolonged disturbing perceptual and emotional experiences, commonly associated with the formation of stuttering behaviors?

This question is best left to speculation. Yet, we can consider, as contended by Shames and Rubin, that walking and speech are fundamentally like other motor performances, and that each skill can be subject to 'momentary and sporadic disruptions' in their motor performances. We might then well assume that the individual's walking, if subjected to sufficiently related traumatic external stimuli, would exhibit chronic disruptions in mobility behaviors.

Genetically specific basic skills, such as walking and speech, develop the respective neurophysiological motor processes using separate organizations of neurons. By comparison, awkward walking and dysfluency behaviors represent similar disturbing neuropsychological experiences. Each behavior depicts the disruptive effects of disturbing perceptions of external influences on the function of specific brain areas, in relation to the proper neurophysiological motor performances for each skill. The neural excitations, reflecting the individual's disturbing perceptions, act upon neural motor cells unrelated to the particular skill, but which can associate with and disrupt the developed neurophysiological motor processes for walking or speech.

We may further reason that movements evident in both disruptive behaviors do not contribute to the proper motor development or performance of the particular affected skill. Awkward walking and dysfluent speech behaviors must therefore represent extraneous motor movements unrelated to the development or performance of these skills. We might characterize these disruptive movements as dysfluent non-walking and dysfluent non-speech motor behaviors.

We are, however, aware of differences between awkward walking and dysfluency behaviors. Although both behaviors result from disruption of the proper neurophysiological motor functions for the skill, episodes of awkward walking are generally much less frequent and of shorter duration. Speech dysfluencies, on the contrary, not only tend to be more often repeated and for longer periods, but also to be regarded as preceding the formation of stuttering behaviors.

Speech dysfluencies, as Shames and Rubin rightly contend, can be 'momentary and sporadic, and thus, not necessarily indicative of stuttering behaviors'. It is, therefore, necessary to identify the major characteristics of the dysfluencies which, more or less, tend to be exhibited in stuttering behaviors. These dysfluencies are referred to as: (1) heightened speech, (2) transitional dysfluencies and (3) stuttering behaviors. The relationships of these states of dysfluent speech (discussed below) should be understood for what they represent, if stuttering behaviors are to be properly dealt with.

Consistent fluent speech movements are the product of repetition and neural plasticity. Subject to their duration and frequency of occurrence, dysfluencies, particularly stuttering, also tend to be produced with relative consistency which suggests that dysfluencies comprise discrete non-speech, rather than speech, movements, and that their transition to stuttering behaviors would tend therefore to follow somewhat similar neurophysiological processes to those involved in the development of fluent speech.

The genetically specific motor neurons for speech cannot, however, perform both fluent speech and dysfluent non-speech motor functions. The motor behaviors for fluent speech and dysfluencies must represent separate neurophysiological motor processes involving different organizations of motor neurons. Intentional stuttering is not a form of non-speech motor behavior. On the contrary, it is a volitional fluent speech display of attempted repetitive dysfluencies.

Changes in the neurophysiological motor processes for the discrete behaviors of a particular skill can be influenced by the individual's positive or negative perceptual responses to external stimuli (Fitts and Patterson, 1964). It should also be noted that, as a result of selective rigidity, the neurophysiological motor functions of specific skills are resistant to changes in other skills or behaviors. Again referring to Goldstein's (1948) statement:

> External influences could selectively affect the formation of specific skills, rather than constitute a generalized disturbance to the formation of a variety of skills.

Specific skills can, however, as Goldstein (1948) also stated, be subject to disruptive influences without incurring changes in their basic functions, as a result of their neural rigidity. This rigidity of neuronal organizations for specific skills enabled the individual to regain his developed walking skills once the disturbing perceptions were removed. We know that stutterers, as for non-stutterers, not only continue to exhibit normal fluent speech in spite of episodes of dysfluency behaviors, but also commonly show no disturbances to other skills.

Paradoxically, stuttering behaviors, formed as discrete neurophysiological non-speech movements, appear to be as similarly subject to the protective functions of neural rigidity as the discrete motor behaviors for fluent speech. Neural rigidity may, consequently, also account for the apparent resistance historically shown in stuttering behaviors to the application of a wide range of professional and pseudo-professional therapy approaches.

The similarities and differences of different dysfluency states are pertinent to neurophysiological and neuropsychological factors touched on earlier, and discussed later. These factors relate to the individual's constant efforts to maintain homeostasis (adjustment to one's self and environment), which Goldstein (1948) maintained was essential for initiating and sustaining actions, skills and behaviors.

> *Comments*: this section has endeavored to provide a somewhat simplified, but rational, basis for the dual-tract motor program for stuttering discussed below. The functional aspects of this two-tract neurophysiological motor program are deemed essential for understanding the neuropsychological factors relevant to the individual's repeated episodes of stuttering behaviors, and the psychosocial approach for treating with these disruptive behaviors.

A chronology for developmental stuttering

The exact chronology for an individual's formation of developmental stuttering is often difficult to determine, because clinical attention is more commonly sought after such behaviors are deemed to have occurred. We may, however, treat this subject as consisting of three general stages. The time frames between these stages will vary and overlap depending on individual experiences, perceptions, emotional responses, maturation, etc. These generalized stages are termed: the pre-dysfluency stage; the transitional dysfluency stage; and the dual-tract motor program stage. These stages can be experienced at ages as early as 2 and 3 years, and up to puberty. There have been reports of an onset of stuttering well into adulthood.

The pre-dysfluency stage

Van Riper, among others, maintains that stuttering often begins with overly concerned parental assessments of the child's early non-fluency behaviors, which are often evident in his normal on-going speech development. Johnson's semantic approach maintained that stuttering starts with the child's self-perception as a stutterer.

Common to both views is the child's confusing perception of such external stimuli, fostered by parents and/or others, which threaten his early inhibited dependence on speech as a primary means for obtaining gratification experiences. As a result of limited experiences, the child usually lacks prior alternative programs of action to cope with these confusing perceptions. The child, therefore, often attempt to do so by heightening, i.e. intensifying, the current manner of his speech, including its non-fluencies.

This display of heightened speech behaviors may be regarded as the pre-dysfluency stage. These behaviors tend to reflect the child's efforts to maintain homeostasis by asserting his speech gratification dependence. The more dominant of these heightened speech behaviors are listed below:

- A noticeable increase in his speech rate.
- Sustained efforts to speak after apparently running out of speech breath, and at times upon inhalation.
- An evident urgency to express himself.
- An apparent increase in the intensity and duration of his non-fluency behaviors: repetitions, oral hesitations, prolongations, mild blockings, etc.
- A seeming tendency to use what may appear to be coping behaviors (starters).

The child's heightened speech behaviors stemmed mostly from his lack of maturity and prior alternative speech experiences (internal programs of action). These factors compound the disturbing attentions directed towards his speech, and his failure to comprehend what is being required of him. The child, however, generally remains eager, self-assertive and uninhibited in his expressive speech behaviors. In spite of his confusion, he usually does not exhibit sustained tensions or related overt negative emotions.

There appears to be a comparable relationship between the child's confused heightened speech behaviors and examples of the awkward walking behaviors provoked by disturbing perceptions of external stimuli. Concerning this similarity, it seemed proper to refer again to the comments of Shames and Rubin (1986):

> . . . not all behaviors that affect the forward flow of speech are indicative of disorganization or disorder. Even the presence of dysfluencies that are indicative of breakdown are not necessarily evidence of a disorder. They may merely be the result of a momentary and sporadic lack of the organization that fluency production requires.

When these conditions persist, however, the child's confusion may become more intensified and disturbing, as he gropes for means to come to adequate terms with the disturbing stimuli. Sustained failure to do so tends to evoke more disturbing perceptions and confused emotions, leading to ever increased heightened speech behaviors, and the progression of this pre-dysfluency stage into the transitional dysfluency stage.

Comments: Van Riper maintained that preventing the child's non-fluency behaviors from developing into more chronic dysfluency behaviors is usually very good. Prevention requires ceasing to reinforce his confusing perceptions and negative responses through improper attention and demands related to his speech needs, and providing proper motivational support for self-expression, with ample speech gratification experiences. Heightened speech behaviors may be mistakenly diagnosed and treated as chronic dysfluency behaviors, leading to negative consequences that have to be borne by the child throughout his life.

The transitional dysfluency stage

Speech is a primary medium through which humans interact and seek gratification from their relationships with others. The child's loss of speech gratification experiences, and his inability to cope with the disturbing stimuli towards his heightened speech, can lead to increased disturbing confusion and related negative emotional states.

Nevertheless, the child attempts to maintain his speech gratification dependence, which has become a primary basis for his homeostasis. His inability to do so may lead to feelings of helplessness and intimidation, which tend to prelude the transition of his heightened speech to chronic dysfluency behaviors (stuttering).

The child's sustained feelings of helplessness and intimidation during this transitional dysfluency stage become evident in his extraneous non-speech motor behaviors, i.e. facial and bodily tensions with distorted movements, as well as avoidance ploys. These non-speech motor behaviors denote his continued lack of proper alternative programs which might gratify his needs and efforts to cope with these discomforting experiences.

Within the latter part of this stage, the child begins to perceive and internalize his feelings of helplessness, frustration and greater uncertainty in his speech efforts. These increased negative emotional states and related behaviors tend to promote traumatic neuropsychological reactions, sufficient to influence the neurophysiological organization and functions of diffused assemblies of non-speech motor neurons within his brain.

This improper activation of these diffused non-speech motor neurons forms the bases for the neurophysiological formation of the child's dysfluencies and related extraneous non-speech behaviors within a secondary non-speech motor program (Fitts, 1973). This secondary non-speech motor program is regarded as fundamental to the dual-tract motor program approach to the formation of developmental stuttering.

In summary: the child's inability to adjust to disturbing external stimuli relating to his speech-dependence needs can result in a loss of speech gratification experiences, confusion, feelings of helplessness and related negative emotional states. The child may, therefore, respond traumatically to these negative emotional states when there is a lack of maturity and/or prior experiences giving him some degree of predictability for coping with these disturbing conditions.

These negative emotional responses can provide the bases for traumatic neuropsychological reactions, such as negative preoccupations and anticipations. These reactions can be disturbed pre-speech SETs which tend to promote not only the formation of developmental stuttering behaviors within a secondary non-speech motor program, but also the individual's repeated episodes of his dysfluency behaviors and their resistance to therapy techniques.

The external stimuli provoking the child's disturbing perceptions, negative emotions and consequent traumatic reactions, which are able effectively to influence organizations of motor neurons, can come in many forms and from many sources. The point here is that stuttering behaviors more often tend to be associated with some form of traumatic speech or speech-related experience.

Comments: in spite of the transition of the child's heightened speech to apparent dysfluency behaviors, the neurophysiological, non-speech motor processes for these behaviors may not, as yet, become perseverated within a secondary motor program (this is discussed in more detail below). With proper handling, therefore, perseveration of these symptomatic stuttering behaviors can be checked. Such handling should be based upon:

1. Avoiding undue attention that may lead to undue preoccupation with his speech and the onset of negative anticipations of the outcome of participating in speech events.
2. Restoring dependence on speech as a readily available means of communicating for speech gratification experiences by providing meaningful opportunities related to the individual's needs and interests.
3. Relieving feelings of helplessness and related negative attitudes and emotions in the use of speech, by providing acceptance and affections without demands on speech.
4. Seeking the early counsel of a qualified speech pathologist if unsure of what to do, or whether problems persist.

The above reflect the critical nature of the transitory dysfluency stage. If, during this stage, the child's pronounced dysfluency behaviors are not prevented from perseverating within a secondary non-speech motor program, they will tend to become neurophysiologically automated as disruptive stuttering behaviors

The dual-tract motor program stage

This stage relates to the neuronal formation of two separate, but associated, neurophysiological motor programs within the brain. These two motor programs consist of:

- A basic motor program for developed fluent speech performances.
- A secondary non-speech motor program containing non-speech movements representing the dysfluency behaviors (stuttering), with the potential to disrupt fluent speech performances.

Some authorities contend that stuttering is an expression of the individual's need to cope with problems he cannot otherwise resolve. Generally, however, stutterers do not intentionally stutter, but rather strive to use their normally developed fluent speech as a readily available means of gratifying their communication needs, free from the personal, social and vocational restrictions that they often experience.

We are well aware that people exhibiting stuttering behaviors do not do so within all speech situations. Nor are they dysfluent on all consonants, syllables, words or even phrases while exhibiting stuttering behaviors. It should be apparent therefore that, in all their efforts to speak, the basic motor program, within which are formed the neurophysiological motor processes for their developed fluent speech, is always being activated.

Furthermore, as noted earlier, the neural assemblies forming the basic motor program for speech cannot produce both the discrete movements for fluent speech and the discrete disruptive movements for stuttering. This would logically imply not only the formation of separate motor programs for each – the individual developed fluent speech and the disruptive non-speech stuttering behaviors – but also that both motor programs tend to be activated during episodes of stuttering.

The following contentions tend to support the formation of dual-tract motor programs:

1. Genetic specificity: neuronal systems possessing the genetic specificity for basic skills, be it walking, reading or speech, do not develop different and conflicting neurophysiological motor processes for performance of the same skill.
2. Brain-scan devices are providing insights into the functions of specific and general areas of the brain. Canadian researchers are currently using positron emission tomography (PET) in studies of the neuronal speech centers with adult stutterers and non-stutterers; they reported:
   (a) Widely diffused brain activity during episodes of stuttering by adult subjects, when not under tranquillizers.
   (b) Consistent neural activity limited primarily to specific speech motor areas within the brain, in tests with adult stutterers performing fluent speech while under tranquillizers.
   (c) Similar patterns of neural activity in specific speech motor areas in tests of adult stutterers under tranquillizers and adult non-stutterers.
   (d) Consistent neural activity within both the specific speech areas and diffused networks of motor cells, during adult episodes of stuttering behaviors. These test results would tend to support the activation of the dual-tract motor programs during episodes of stuttering behaviors.
3. The relative consistency in the individual's performances of both his developed fluent speech and involuntary stuttering behaviors. This strongly suggests separate closed circuit neural memory tracts for the neurophysiological formation and activation of these two different behaviors within separate motor programs located in different areas of the brain.

4. Neural loops comprising closed circuit memory tracts for a particular skill, as a function of neural rigidity, cannot retain two conflicting motor programs. Goldstein (1939) stressed that the neural rigidity of the motoneurons resisted disruptive influences on the normal neurophysiological processes for the performance of developed basic skills and behaviors.

   Neural rigidity of the motoneurons can work both ways, for positive as well as negative behaviors. Considering the stubborn resistance of stuttering behaviors to remedial techniques, neural rigidity may well apply to stuttering behaviors. This would give further support to their formation within a secondary motor program.
5. Goldstein's reference to the selective effects of external influences on motor performances of specific basic skills is noted in the relative consistency of the person's stuttering behaviors in disrupting the flow of his fluent speech, rather than other aspects of his speech skill.
6. Recent studies of brain functioning reported that the learning of a skill progressively lessens the areas of the brain required for mediating its performance (*Time*, June 1992). The formation of dual motor programs is further supported by the contention of the Lurias (Luria, 1966a) that post-birth experiences continue to affect the structure and functions of organizations of neural cells within the brain.

The basic motor program for speech: general areas and functions

> The specific speech areas of the brain are still subject to question, and in need of extensive research.
>
> *Love and Webb (1986)*

By selective use of some of the material written about the brain, and spiced with reasoned speculation, I have attempted to provide a general overview of the areas involved in the formation and activation of the motor programs relative to both developed fluent speech and disruptive stuttering behaviors.

The young child's formation of a basic motor program for speech is essential for the normal neurophysiological development and consistent performances of this basic communication skill. Rosenthal (1977) regarded the transition of children's egocentric, self-stimulating vocalizations (i.e. babbling and jargon) into intelligible words and sentences, suggestive of the early formation of consistent motor speech patterns, as indicative of a basic motor program for speech.

Positron emission tomography studies, referred to earlier, showed that speech areas of the brain have extensive interacting neural–fiber connections with related intellect, perceptual emotional faculties, and gross and fine motor centers primarily within the frontal and temporal lobes. These connections to Hebb (1959) suggested closed circuit feedback loops for memory functions associated with the higher cortical levels in the brain. There are also collateral, neuromotor and spindle-loop connections with the cranial nerve system, which innervate the muscles of speech production.

Keele (1968) defined the human brain as consisting of general neuronal systems, and subgroup neurons, contained within several cortical levels, and lower neuronal centers. He applied his functional descriptions of these to all forms of motor skills. They therefore apply to the neurophysiological motor processes for speech performances.

Keele stated that the specific and related brain areas for speech skills interrelate through the general neuronal systems and subgroup neurons. These neural relationships provide for interactions between speech and related neurons within each brain level, and for drawing upon the functions of other brain levels to complement the functional use, as well as the formation of the speech skills.

The general neuronal systems for speech consist of multiple assemblies of neurons within the cortical lobes of the brain. These neuronal systems contain subgroup neurons, which usually function as neural junctions and triggering mechanisms for transmitting sensory excitations to activate the larger general speech neurons. The speech neurons have the potential for preferential plasticity, which enables them to be more readily activated by sensory excitations related to their speech function.

Subgroup neurons are preferentially sensitive as triggering mechanisms to stimulation by sensory excitations. Their considerably lower levels of neural–synaptic resistance enables them to monitor the flow of sensory excitations for passage to the speech neurons for motor speech performances. Subgroup neurons are particularly sensitive to sensory excitations from the perceptory systems, which in turn are very responsive to external stimuli. The subgroup neurons are therefore of special significance in the formation and functions of the dual tract motor programs for speech.

The assemblies of speech neurons are likened to digital systems, which can be programmed to store, organize and retrieve sensory information within closed circuit memory tracts. These processes relate to the levels of resistance these neurons establish for preferential activation by sensory excitations representing specific speech functions.

It is apparent from the above that the formation of a basic motor program for speech requires preferential passage of the perceptual– motor excitations for speech functions to the speech neurons. Preferential passage depends, however, on the compatible interplay between the functions of the speech neurons and the individual's perceptions of his speech experiences, which depend greatly on external stimuli.

The sequence of events leading to the formation of the basic motor program for speech begins with the child's speech gratification experiences, which motivate and reinforce his earliest vocalizations. The sensorimotor movements of these vocalizations are transmitted, in the form of neural excitations, to subgroup neurons for passage across the neurosynaptic connectors to the speech neurons.

Repeated stimulations of the speech neurons by the neural excitations, representing the motor patterns of the child's vocalizations resulting from neural plasticity, lower their neural–synaptic resistance levels; they thus become more prone activation and formation of basic automated neurophysiological motor processes within a basic motor program for speech. These levels of synaptic resistance therefore mediate the functional activations of the speech neurons. The automation of the motor processes for speech enables the child to speak without the need to attend consciously to how the incremental speech movements are to be performed.

Complementary interplay between the child's genetic specificity for speech and the perceptual responses to external stimuli can influence the stability of his speech SETs (Goldstein, 1948). These SETs relate the status of the child's readiness to act, i.e. to speak. Stable speech SETs enable the child to act volitionally and perform synchronously the temporal sequences of the neurophysiological motor processes for his intended speech movements, which are formed and automated within the basic motor program for speech.

In summary: speech gratification experiences, through reinforcement of the child's dependence on speech, serve to motivate its usage, and thus promotes the preferential activation of the speech neurons and the automation of the neurophysiological motor speech processes within the basic motor program for speech. The developing consistency of the child's speech, resulting from automation of neurophysiological motor processes, coupled with the rigidity of the genetic specificity of the speech neurons, suggested to Fitts and Patterson (1964):

> . . . a functional unity encompassed within specific areas of the brain, i.e. a basic motor-program for speech.

A secondary motor program for non-speech stuttering behaviors: brain areas and functions

Stuttering behaviors, as noted earlier, are generated as non-speech neurophysiological motor processes, with the potential to disrupt the forward flow of an individual's developed fluent speech. We have also noted that the non-speech motor processes for stuttering behaviors cannot be produced within the basic motor program for speech, but requires a secondary non-speech motor program.

Young children generally have little need to attend cognitively to the early development or proficiency of their speech performances. They tend in their immaturity to lack sufficient cognitive skills and internal programs of action, which might enable them to effect the necessary degree of control over their developing speech performances. Luria (1966b) maintained that for an individual to change his performances of a skill requires:

- The crucial powers for recognizing reality: the ability to cognitively perceive and selectively mediate one's performance as influenced by prior experiences.
- Internal programs of action: alternative behaviors of a particular skill, learned from previous experiences, which may enable the person to act selectively to change his performances.

The child, unable to cope properly with disturbing perceptions of external demands relating to his speech performances and needs, may experience varying states of confusion, helplessness, intimidation and related negative emotions. He may thus be subjected to traumatic neuropsychological reactions, which can influence disruptive functional changes within organizations of neurons in his developing brain. These functional neuronal changes, caused by factors such as selective rigidity, generally involve the motor performances of specific skills, such as speech.

Other factors, such as genetic specificity, neural rigidity and automation, tend to protect the neurophysiological motor processes of the child's developed fluent speech from change. Consequently, the neural excitations reflecting the non-speech movements of his dysfluencies and related extraneous coping behaviors, and traumatic reactions, will not be allowed passage to the speech neurons at the subgroup neurons because of incompatibility

These incompatible non-speech neural excitations may either dissipate on being resisted passage or be shunted by the subgroup neurons to diffuse, peripheral, non-speech, motoneurons within subcortical areas of the brain. Athough this shunting action may result in other forms of behavioral disorders, it is central to the formation of the secondary non-speech motor program and the stuttering behaviors.

This shunting reflects functional brain disorganization within this peripheral network of diffused motoneurons. In this regard, however, the formation of the secondary non-speech motor program, and the neurophysiological non-speech motor processes representing stuttering behaviors, is fairly similar to the formation of the basic motor program and the neurophysiological motor processes for fluent speech movements. These diffused motoneurons likewise establish levels of neural resistance that are preferentially receptive to the disruptive non-speech motor excitations.

These networks of diffused motor cells are deemed to be within the subcortical levels of the brain, and comprise the main neuronal organizations for the secondary non-speech motor program. These networks have neural associations with the cranial nerves, upper pyramidal tract motoneurons, as well as emotional collaterals within the pre-motor speech areas of the frontal lobes. This allows transmission and reception of neural impulses flowing between the CNS and receptor organs within the speech and related body mechanisms

These networks have collateral neural associations with many upper body gross muscle systems consisting of afferent (sensory) and efferent (motor) nerves comprising fusimotor fibers. These nerve fibers function as pathways for activating movements, and as a servomechanism system operating by means of stretch reflex loops. In his reference to the interactions of these collateral neural associations, Milner (1970) commented:

> Input instructions determine the result independently of the conditions at the muscles involved. The servo-mechanism allows this achievement without requiring storage of an impossibly large number of alternate sets of instructions at the highest level.

The functions of the stretch reflex loops, servomechanism and the lower subcortical positions of these diffused motoneurons would tend to account for the relative consistency of the involuntary patterns of the individual's stuttering behaviors. Also, the spasm movements common to involuntary stuttering behaviors suggest possible neural associations with stretch reflexes and synergistic gross muscle systems (Chusid, 1973).

In summary, stuttering behaviors are represented as disruptive, neurophysiological, non-speech movements formed within and imposed by a secondary non-speech motor program on the stutterer's basic motor program for speech. The secondary non-speech motor program is regarded as encompassing diffuse networks of subcortical motoneurons.

The secondary motor program is activated by a sequence of factors, starting with his disturbing perceptions and emotional responses to preoccupations about negative anticipations towards particular speech events, which disturbed the stability of his pre-speech readiness SETs, and provoked the activating traumatic neuropsychological reactions.

Comments: the notion of dual-tract neurophysiologically formed motor programs, fostered by neuropsychological stimuli, would tend to negate the general belief that stuttering behaviors indicate the disorganization of speech neurons within the brain. In support of this negation, we noted that the neuronal organization for the neurophysiological motor processes of fluent speech are protected by factors, such as genetic specificity, selective neural rigidity and automation. Consequently, the neuronal assemblies for speech do not become disorganized, but rather subject to disruptive episodes in their developed performances.

It was not intended to support the dual-tract motor programs for stuttering by overwhelming readers with a deluge of neurology. I only wanted to depict the complexity of these dual motor tracts, which comprise the bicameral formation of two incompatible neurophysiological motor programs, within different, but interconnected, areas of the brain. These dual-tract motor programs are deemed to be consistent with the neuropsychological approach to developmental stuttering.

It is more than an exercise in semantics to contend that stuttering behaviors, subject to certain conditions, directly deprive the individual of the ready availability of his organized and automated neurophysiological basic motor program for fluent speech. This distinction is deemed important, not only for understanding stuttering, but perhaps more so for treating these repeated behaviors.

Chapter 5
The neuropsychological bases for stuttering behaviors

In the previous chapter, attention was drawn to stuttering behaviors which, as disruptive neurophysiological non-speech motor processes, are formed within a secondary non-speech motor program. These non-speech motor processes, evident as stuttering behaviors, do not inhibit the development of speech, nor are they indicative of changes in the form of the individual's developed speech. Rather, stuttering behaviors are seen as episodes of dysfluency behavior which inhibit the ready availability of developed speech, by disrupting the forward flow of its synchronous movements.

The performances of motor programs for particular skills and behaviors, also noted, can be mediated only by the neuropsychological influences of the executive (master) program (Fitts and Redford, 1966). Stuttering consists of relatively discrete non-speech behaviors (Van Riper, 1973), formed within a secondary non-speech motor program, which are subject to the mediating neuropsychological influences of the executive program, as for other skills and behaviors. Stuttering behaviors, although disruptive to fluent speech, are nevertheless formed unrelated to both speech development and its performance.

Stuttering is a complex neuropsychological phenomenon. This notion relates to neuropsychological variables, such as anticipation, perceptions, gratifications, attitudes and emotional states. These variables, depending on the extent of their positive or negative status, can effectively influence the manner of the executive (master) motor program's activation of the neurophysiological processess within the dual-tract motor programs for both fluent speech and stuttering behaviors respectively.

The above notion is consistent with the contention of the Lurias (Luria, 1966a) that neuropsychological factors can effect negative, as well as positive, changes in the neuronal functions of skills and behaviors. Consequently, when these neuropsychological variables are positive, stutterers can be expected to exhibit considerable, if not total, reduction in dysfluency behaviors. When negative, these variables tend to influence the severity and frequency of the stuttering behaviors.

Anticipation

One of the more dominant neuropsychological variables closely associated with stuttering behaviors is anticipation, defined as:

1. Anticipating or being anticipated.
2. Something anticipated or expected.
3. Foreknowledge; presentiment.
4. What is likely or desired to occur.

Anticipation may also relate to actions, such as to anticipate, to expect, to await, to depend upon, to predict (*Webster's Dictionary*, 1970).

G.K. Chesterton (1985) observed:

> We may all, at one time or another, have experienced more pleasure from our anticipations of things desired, than from obtaining the things anticipated.

For stutterers, however, anticipation of the desired outcome of their efforts to produce fluent speech, more often as not leads to experiences that are less pleasurable than their desired anticipation.

Non-stutterers and stutterers tend to differ in their respective desired anticipations regarding their speech efforts. Non-stutterers more commonly anticipate gratification through their use of speech, rather than from the manner of speech performances. More often, stutterers are considerably more preoccupied with their efforts to speak fluently, as a source of gratification. What factors, present or absent within certain speech experiences, tend to promote the conditions that trigger stuttering behaviors – awaiting like 'fifth columns', ready to disrupt the neurophysiological motor processes for the stutterers' developed fluent speech?

Readiness SETs for speech

Stutterers are often presented with a dilemma between anticipations. Successful speech experiences serve to promote positive anticipations towards certain speech situations, whereas unsuccessful speech experiences foster and sustain negative anticipations towards other speech events. As anticipations generally precede active speech, the stutterers' positive or negative anticipations will often affect the outcome of their participation in speech situations, by influencing their readiness SETs to participate.

Goldstein (1948) defined a readiness SET as: 'the act of ordering the body into a state of readiness to perform specific functions'. Goldstein's concept on readiness SETs to act was based on his work with soldiers afflicted with head injuries. He held that thinking is an act, a form of movement, which can stimulate chronaxie (electrical excitations of muscle or nerve tissue) changes throughout the body. Thoughts of a pretty woman can arouse changes in chronaxie excitations at a man's toes, cheeks and elsewhere. He also maintained that, as the nervous system is never at rest, it is always in a constant state of neural excitation, which provides the organism with its readiness SETs to act. This might be likened to a car idling in neutral position: ready to be set in motion with activation of the clutch–gear system.

Goldstein regarded the act of anticipating as an abstract form of thinking, although nevertheless movement. As such, the individual's acts of anticipating his participation in speech performances could generate subliminal (below threshold of awareness or action), chronaxie, sensory excitations to the speech motor centers. The motoneurons within these centers would therefore subliminally energize the muscle systems for speech, thereby placing them in a readiness SET to perform speech, but without activating movements of the speech mechanisms.

The stutterer's anticipations towards speech events tend, however, to be subject to preconditioned influences of negative neuropsychological components, such as disturbing perceptions, uncertain attitudes and emotional responses. These components generate ambiguous sensory excitations, which preferentially pass to diffused networks of non-speech motor neurons comprising the secondary non-speech motor program; here the neurophysiological motor processes for the individual's stuttering behaviors are formed. These activated non-speech motoneurons thus subliminally energize non-speech muscles, thereby disturbing the individual's readiness SETs to perform speech, without actual movements of his speech mechanisms.

The above may be illustrated by the athlete assuming the pre-racing readiness SET in his positive anticipation to run to win. In effect, the muscle systems for the required bodily racing movements are being subliminally stimulated, but without being activated into motion. His mental and bodily systems are therefore placed in a readiness SET status to respond to the starter's gun. At the sound of the gun the unity of his mind and body is fluidly set into motion; the racer is off and running to fulfill his anticipations of winning the gold.

The runner might, however, become preoccupied with distracting perceptions, doubts and emotional responses. The ambiguous sensory excitations generated by these distracting neuropsychological stimuli could disturb his mental and motor readiness SETs for running. These disturbances to this readiness SET disrupt the functional unity of his mental and bodily systems to act in fullest concert with each other, thereby jeopardizing the desired gratifications (rewards) anticipated from his racing performance.

This stability of readiness SETs for speech is, in large part, the result of the relative automation of the neurophysiological motor processes for speech formed within its basic motor program. This enables us to attend more to our intentions (seeking gratifications) from our speech efforts, with little conscious attention towards performing the movements required for its phonatory production.

Furthermore, this dependence on speech gratification experiences enabled the young child not only to develop speech, but also to reinforce and maintain its use as a primary motivational power, which, for stutterers, becomes more or less a restricted power. This relative restriction is regarded as a dominant factor in repeated occurrences of stutterers' involuntary dysfluency behaviors.

The stability of our readiness SETs for speech, as with other social skills and behaviors, closely relates to our perceptions, attitudes and emotional responses towards external stimuli. We are communal–social creatures, ever conscious of the need to seek and anticipate gratification from external sources through our dependence on speech. Disturbances to the stability of the stutterers' readiness SETs for speech are, thus, also fostered by preoccupations with negative anticipations towards the social consequences of exposing their dysfluency behaviors.

Goldstein also regarded thinking as a form of inner speech which is therefore subject to the neuropsychological and neurophysiological functions related directly to actual phonated speech. During acts of inner speech, the motoneurons for speech stimulate the muscle systems for speech subliminally, in a manner corresponding directly to the synchronous temporal sequences of the individual's unvoiced inner speech phonatory speech patterns, but without activating movements of the speech mechanisms. Goldstein contended that similar patterns of subliminal chronaxie stimulations occur during silent reading.

When the stutterer's thoughts (inner speech) are preoccupied with negative anticipations towards his speech efforts and/or the non-gratifying consequences, disturbing perceptions, attitudes and emotional responses tend to become more manifest and traumatically reactive. These neuropsychological components and variables may therefore not only contribute towards the instability of his readiness SETs for speech before performance, but also predispose the individual into a readiness SET for stuttering.

In summary: readiness SETs for speech are subject to the influences of the neuropsychological components comprising the executive (master) program. These components relate to the individual's perceptions, attitudes and emotional responsess. Disturbances of these components can negatively influence the stutterer's anticipations. Preoccupation with negative anticipations generates ambiguous distracting neural excitations, which can disturb the stability of his readiness SETs for performing desired fluent speech; these then contribute towards triggering repeated activations of his disruptive stuttering behaviors, formed within a secondary non-speech motor program.

Coping adjustment methods, speech-related struggles and associated stuttering behaviors

The early development of speech did not depend on the child's preoccupation with concerns for its proper usage or phonatory development. These aspects of speech depended more on the child's imitative responses, motivated and reinforced by gratification experiences. To make the child unduly preoccupied with his speech can disrupt its primary motivational power (Piaget, 1968) as a ready means for fulfilling his natural inclination for gratification experiences. To frustrate the child's need for gratification experiences may lead to a form of behavioral disorder, possibly developmental stuttering.

The literature on stuttering seems to accord little importance and little attention to the close relationship between certain behavioral characteristics and stuttering. On the contrary, coping adjustment methods, speech-related struggles and associated stuttering behaviors warrant proper attention because they contribute, not only to the stutterers' repertoire of dysfluency behaviors, but also to the repeated occurrences of these disruptive behaviors.

The preoccupations of stutterers with the outcome and consequences of their speech efforts are evident in their tendency to employ coping adjustment methods. These are usually in the form of self-manipulating or distracting techniques, generally referred to as starters or speech crutches. These techniques are volitionally employed to enable the users to begin and/or sustain their speech efforts, by controlling, avoiding or suppressing their stuttering behaviors. The variety of such techniques, ranging from weird to seemingly practical, might well equal the total number of stutterers, in spite of considerable overlap in the usage of certain of these coping methods.

Successful speech experiences with the use of coping methods would tend to promote their continued usage, and more positive anticipations towards participating in speech events. On the other hand, we would expect stutterers to stop using these techniques when they cease to enhance their efforts to speak with relative fluency, as well as viewing the use of coping adjustment methods with somewhat negative anticipations. Yet, coping methods like drugs can become addictive, supported irrationally in spite of their diminishing gratification, and they can foster additional problems.

Although coping adjustment methods, starters and related distraction techniques or devices may provide some initial relief from the tyranny of stuttering behaviors, the benefits of such methods tend to be short-lived. Paradoxically, the initial speech gratification experiences with coping methods tend to diminish with usage, rather than reinforce their seeming benefits as speech aids. Furthermore, the continued usage of coping methods, past their diminishing values to enhance fluent speech, is indicative of the user's vain attempts to regain the initial benefits.

That hope may defy logic is evident in the general persistence of stutterers, striving for fluency, to use particular coping methods in spite of their diminished value as speech aids. Continued reliance on such coping methods tends to heighten feelings of helplessness and related disturbing emotional responses, which, reflecting their lack of alternative means to act inadvertently increase the individual's dependence on the methods. This dependence is evident in their more intensive efforts to use the failing coping methods, which become speech-related struggles.

Coping adjustment methods tend to lose their values as speech aids, mainly because these methods generally do not relate to either the neuropsychological or the neurophysiological processes that promote normal speech development or its performance. On the contrary, these methods tend to be in opposition to the essential processes for speech. Coping adjustment methods tend to be extraneous, non-speech, behavioral artifacts, by which the users attempt to circumvent, through self-manipulative techniques, their stuttering behaviors to enable them to gain ready access to their developed fluent speech processes.

The speech-related struggles, generated as perceptual–motor excitations to the subneurons for speech, are not allowed passage to the speech neurons mainly because of (1) neural synaptic plasticity and resistance, and (2) the relative compatibility of these behavioral artifacts with the individual's non-speech stuttering behaviors. Instead, these non-speech excitations are preferentially shunted to the diffused networks of non-speech motor neurons comprising the secondary motor program for stuttering behaviors.

Within the secondary motor program, the behavioral artifacts are integrated within the neurophysiological motor processes for stuttering behaviors to become involuntary additions to the individual's repertoire, as associated stuttering behaviors. I regard these added stuttering behaviors as the involuntary behavioral residues of volitional coping adjustment methods, which have become part of the problem, rather than contributing to its solution.

The transition of the individual's coping adjustment methods into speech-related struggles, and their subsequent fixation into involuntary asssociated stuttering behaviors, suggests that such methods tend to promote the disturbing neuropsychological and neurophysiological conditions in a similar fashion; these not only can lead to stuttering behaviors, but also to the repeated occurrences of these behaviors.

Coping methods require constant preoccupation with the manipulatory functions of their usage and with the anticipated results. With the diminishing of the speech gratification experiences provided initially by these methods, the user's dependence on speech tends to be transferred to the coping methods. This would account for the persistent use of these methods, as speech-related struggles, in spite of their lost benefits as speech aids.

Stutterers need not comprehend the neuropsychological complexities of their increasing preoccupation with the inadequacies of the coping methods in forming negative anticipations that are counterproductive to their intended objectives. Their persistent speech-related struggles to salvage the diminishing benefits of the coping methods are indicative of disturbing perceptions, feelings of helplessness, uncertain attitudes and negative emotions. These neuropsychological components contribute towards the instability of the readiness SETs necessary for performing speech, which tends to lead to increased frequency of stuttering behaviors.

The child's heightened speech behaviors might be considered as early coping adjustment methods. It is doubtful, however, whether he is preoccupied with negative anticipations regarding the status of his speech. More probably he cannot fully comprehend what is being rejected in his speech or what is expected of him and lacks alternative programs. His coping efforts would therefore tend to be directed towards avoiding the discomforting feelings about the loss of his previous dependence on speech as a source of gratification experiences.

During the transition from heightened speech behaviors to more chronically exhibited dysfluencies, the child may appear to be using coping adjustment methods, which are usually related to reflexive facial grimacing and bodily tensions. These behaviors tend, however, to be more indicative of his efforts towards retaining his speech gratification dependence, rather then volitional techniques for self-administration of his dysfluencies. Nor is the child beset with negative anticipations regarding the outcome of his more heightened dysfluency behaviors.

Brutten, and Wingate, among others, in spite of references to coping adjustment behaviors, apparently do not consider them typical stuttering behaviors, which they imply consist mainly of the involuntary classical stuttering symptoms. Brutten, in this regard, offered the following comment:

> The coping adjustments behaviors that are seemingly used to avoid and escape speech difficulties are not typically considered to be stuttering by those who stutter.

This comment appears somewhat difficult to accept, because stutterers more commonly tend to employ coping adjustment methods, volitionally or not, to avoid or escape speech difficulties and the social and/or vocational consequences of exhibiting stuttering behaviors. If this is so, then it might similarly be reasoned that:

> A person's concerns for coping with his crippled legs are not significantly related to the means he might employ to off-set the limited mobility his condition imposes upon his walking needs.

A person's preoccupation with certain characteristics of his handicap may foster disturbing self-perceptions and attitudes, which can impose greater handicaps, and resistance to therapy and proper adjustment, than the extent of the disability itself. Could not the omission or negation of certain unpleasant aspects of the handicap also limit proper diagnostic understanding by overlooking the true extent to which these aspects contribute to its severity, and the limitations or deprivations of life experiences? Furthermore, would not omission or negation of these aspects frustrate therapy efforts which might otherwise achieve beneficial results?

I do not regard stuttering as a handicap, but rather a conditional behavioral problem. Yet, there appear to be good reasons to assert that the diagnostic and remedial consequences of omission or negation of certain behaviors, as stated above, might well apply to stuttering. To start with:

> Do not the more overtly obvious, and perhaps ungainly, facial, head and bodily behaviors exhibited during stuttering stem from the individual's coping methods to avoid and escape displaying such behaviors?

I have worked with many adult stutterers who regarded the removal or reduction of their overt struggling behaviors as significant therapy successes.

Proper diagnostic and therapy assessments consider the total patterns of the person's stuttering behaviors, which foster the individual's negative self-perceptions, preoccupations, attitudes, anticipations, emotional responses, etc. These negative neuropsychological components relate, as much or more, to an inability to cope with overt stuttering behaviors as to these behaviors themselves. Furthermore, his inability to cope with these negative neuropsychological components contributes greatly to the instability of his readiness SETs for speech, which serves towards promoting the frequency, and thus the severity, of his repeated episodes of stuttering behaviors.

Comments: to disregard the significance of the stutterer's use and the consequences of employing coping adjustment methods to promote fluent speech overlooks both the diagnostic and the remedial importance of his speech-related struggles. Experiencing the loss of the early benefits of coping adjustment methods may not only alter the characteristics of the individual's stuttering behaviors, but also promote negative anticipations and resistance towards more potentially beneficial therapy methods.

There are indications within the literature of a somewhat moot controversy about the objectives of stutterers in their use of coping adjustment methods. Some authors infer that stutterers rely upon such methods to control, suppress, escape, etc., stuttering behaviors to avoid speech difficulties. Other authors contend that stutterers resort to coping methods primarily to speak with fluency. These two views are as debatable as attempting to discern whether a cup is half-full or half-empty.

Yet, might it not be more motivating and productive to promote optimistic anticipations towards therapy methods? Would this not reinforce the ready availability of clients' developed fluent-speech, rather than fostering preoccupations with negative anticipatory reactions towards escaping or avoiding speech difficulties? Socrates might have resolved this by commenting:

The joy to be anticipated by ceasing to beat one's head against a wall, is the pleasurable release from the pains of doing so.

Anticipation and readiness SETs, and de-differentiation of functions

Goldstein's (1939) concepts about de-differentiation of functions are based on his extensive work with soldiers who incurred head injuries during the Second World War, and with aphasic patients for many years thereafter. He determined that aphasic patients exhibited a generalized breakdown, not only in symbolic language, but also in the performances of its instrumentalities, such as speech, writing, drawing, reading, etc.

Goldstein referred to this breakdown as dedifferentiation of functions, by which he could define performance changes resulting from brain injuries within the context of the effects such injuries have on the whole person. Goldstein defined dedifferentiation of functions as the generalized systematic disintegration of language and speech processes, which he related to the individual's inability to maintain proper abstract attitudes related to performance of language–speech skills.

Although some authorities related dysfluency behaviors to neurological anomalies, I know of no neuropathological (organic) causal relationship between aphasic symptoms and developmental stuttering behaviors. Nor do stutterers exhibit a generalized breakdown in language and its instrumentalities, as do aphasic subjects. Yet, in my work with stutterers and aphasic subjects, certain similarities about dedifferentiation of functions for motor speech modalities, common to aphasic symptoms, also appear to be present in stutterers, but only during their episodes of stuttering behaviors.

> *Comments*: we should note the above distinction because it is contended that the neuropsychological conditions for activating repeated episodes of stuttering behaviors can begin before the individual actually vocalizes his intended speech performance.

Anticipatory reactions, and readiness SETs for speech, are subject to influences of the executive (master) program neuropsychological components, which can affect the differentiation of speech functions. These functions include, among other things, the selection and categorization of symbolic representations of speech with the perceptual–motor movements in relation to the production of the individual's automated developed speech. According to Goldstein (1948), these functions require the proper ordering of readiness SETs for the neurophysiological components of the motor speech processes to act uniformly.

The brain is constantly in motion to maintain readiness SETs for various modalities: sensorimotor, mobility, intellect, memory, etc., as well as to sustain the functions of bodily life-support systems. This, however, also enables organically damaged neurons to energize (irritate) neighboring undamaged neurons continuously, as well as distant neurons relative to specific functions of the damaged neurons. This irritation to undamaged neurons disturbs the neurophysiological stability of aphasic subjects' readiness SETs to act by producing a constant distracting backgound of neural noise, disruptive to the differentiation processes of aphasic subjects.

Although the conditions for stuttering tend to start the stutterer's actual display of dysfluency behaviors, the time periods for these episodes may vary depending on the particular circumstances. These conditions tend to begin with the individual's relatively traumatic neuropsychological reactions to preoccupations with disturbing perceptions, uncertain attitudes and emotional responses towards participation in particular speech events, which foster negative anticipations.

With the brain in constant motion, these neuropsychological reactions generate extraneous sensory excitations which stimulate (irritate) diffused assemblies of non-speech motoneurons. This disturbing stimulation of these motoneurons causes them to be indiscriminately energized, and therefore disruptive to the stability of the readiness SETs required for actively performing their developed speech.

Dedifferentiation (breakdown) of the following functions related to motor speech performances, although common to aphasic symptoms, also appears to be present to some degree during individuals' actual display of stuttering behaviors. The breakdown of these functions relates mainly, as noted above, to neuronal instability, which disturbed the readiness SETs required for:

1. Establishing readiness SETs for speech acts.
2. Establishing readiness SETs for new speech acts within sudden changing circumstances. This relates very closely to the inability to maintain stable neural thresholds.
3. Shifting from one aspect of a speech event to another. This affects the determination of the figure–ground relationships. There are reports of functional disturbances to the visual and auditory modalities during stuttering behaviors (Curlee and Perkins, 1984).

   Dysfunctions of these behaviors relate to lability (instability) of neural thresholds, rises in neural thresholds and retardation of sensory excitations, resulting in decreased reception, and increased reaction time.
4. Identifying and selecting alternative programs of action, which may enable the individual to alter his disrupted behaviors. Often, this may be only to stop his behaviors volitionally.
5. Difficulty detaching his ego from the influences of external speech-related stimuli resulting from exaggerated perceptual attachment and responses to these stimuli. This would also relate to difficulty exercising volitional control during stuttering behaviors

The relative similarities in dedifferentiation of the functions of the above behaviors, common to aphasic symptoms, and during stuttering behaviors have different causes. This suggests that, with regard to stuttering, specific neuronal functions can be effectively disturbed by external influences, so as to produce episodes of involuntary motor behaviors disruptive to the performances of developed speech. The implications of these relationships further suggest certain possible fallacies which may relate to current approaches for treating stuttering behaviors (discussed in Chapter 6).

In summary, negative anticipations, as a form of inner speech, fostered by preoccupation with negative anticipations, can evoke neuropsychological reactions, which activate subliminal excitations that are disturbing to the individual's readiness SETs for speech, without initiating movements of the speech mechanisms. It seems evident that, without maintaining consistent stable speech SETs, stutterers are not in a prepared state of readiness to speak fluently. In effect, stutterers have begun to stutter *before* producing phonated speech.

Aphasic symptoms are the result of neuropathological brain damage, whereas stuttering behaviors are not; this book maintains that the latter are the result of functional neuropsychological disturbances. There appear, however, to be similarities between certain generalized aphasic symptom and stuttering behaviors, with regard to disturbances to readiness SETs for speech motor functions. It was further suggested that such disturbances may not only promote repeated episodes of stuttering behaviors, but also inhibit beneficial therapy results.

A working definition for developmental stuttering

As the basic causes for a behavioral disorder, seemingly as complex as stuttering, are as yet considered to be unknown, it might help to provide a rational overview for this attempt to form a working definition. It is contended that the stutterer's preoccupations with his uncertain dependence on speech leads to negative emotional responses to disturbing perceptions of external stimuli (conditions), which evoke traumatic neuropsychological reactions, manifested as stuttering behaviors, that disrupt the forward flow of his developed speech.

Although the causes for stuttering are regarded as unknown, we do know enough about stuttering to refrain from labeling its behaviors as a speech disorder or handicap. To be labeled as a speech disorder is a misrepresentation of stuttering. To treat stuttering as a handicap is to misunderstand and promote the negative psychosocial consequences which are too often imposed on the stutterer's personal, social and vocational experiences. Stuttering is rather a psychosocial behavioral problem (or disorder), which reflects the breakdown in the on-going interactions between the individual and his socioenvironments.

The classical stuttering symptoms are regarded to comprise mainly involuntary single or combined audible and silent repetitions, or prolongations of short dysrythmic speech elements. These symptoms are evident in sounds, syllables and words, with varying states of phonatory and/or articulatory tonic and/or clonic blockings of the vocal or oral mechanisms (Wingate, 1975). These symptoms are usually the earliest indications of the formation of chronic stuttering behaviors.

Associated stuttering behaviors generally involve single or combinations of mild to extreme extraneous, involuntary facial, head and bodily movements, which tend to accentuate the classical symptoms. These behaviors are often formed as the residual by-products of the individual's speech-related struggles to maintain the use of coping adjustment methods, such as starters, which enable the stutterer to perform his developed fluent speech more readily. Coping methods generally lose their seemingly initial values as speech aids.

The neurophysiology of stuttering relates to formation of dual-tract motor programs; a basic motor program for developed speech and a secondary non-speech motor program for the disruptive stuttering behaviors. Consequently, each motor program is formed within different organizations of motoneurons as different neurophysiological motor processes, within different areas of the brain. Collateral neural associations between these motor programs enable the stuttering behaviors, comprising extraneous non-speech motor processes, to disrupt the forward flow of the individual's developed speech.

The formation of dual-tract motor programs relates to the neuropsychological concept that external stimuli, whether positive or negative, can effect changes in the functions of neural organizations within the brain. The child's disturbing perceptions of external speech-related stimuli evoke traumatic emotional responses (confusion, feelings of helplessness), which generate ambiguous sensory excitations to non-speech motoneurons within the brain. Ambiguous excitation of these motoneurons disrupts the neural stability of the child's readiness SETs to perform his developing, or developed, speech, which can, in effect, place him in a preconditioned status of readiness to stutter.

Stutterers, within particular speech situations, tend to be preoccupied with disturbing perceptions towards the uncertain outcomes of their dependence on speech, which evoke negative anticipations. These preoccupations not only contribute towards the instability of his readiness SETs to perform speech, but also provoke traumatic neuropsychological reactions which activate the repeated episodes of involuntary disruptive non-speech dysfluency behaviors, formed within the secondary motor program.

Comments: it has been long apparent that therapy methods, which attempt to apply primarily mechanistic/manipulative techniques intended to control, suppress, avoid, etc., his stuttering behaviors, have at best gained limited consistent beneficial results. Considering the above, it would seem logical that more beneficial and consistent therapy results could be obtained by treating the conditions, which tend to promote the individual's repeated episodes of stuttering behaviors.

Chapter 6
A psychosocial approach for treating developmental stuttering

If a thing is worth doing, it is worth doing, even if poorly.

G.K. Chesterton (1985)

I might add to Mr Chesterton's comment, '. . . unless it might be done better'. It is certain that Mr Chesterton implied this addition in his worthy comment. The readers can, as I can, think of many things today that are well worth doing, that are being done poorly, but that can be done much better. Although this book strongly contends that providing therapy for stutterers is well worth doing, it also expresses concerns that the current efforts to do so might be done better.

This book intends no direct or implied negative criticisms of the thousands of speech pathologists and allied therapists endeavoring to provide the best beneficial therapy for stutterers. Nor does it rile against the somewhat tolerant indifference of the general public towards stutterers. It does, however, question the apparent rigidity and limitations of current therapy approaches, which attempt to treat stuttering as if its dysfluency behaviors can be treated separately from the psychosocial problems that sustain these disruptive behaviors.

It seemed appropriate to begin by noting again the more dominant past and current methods for treating stuttering behaviors:

- Restrictive oral devices: to limit tongue and jaw movements; often painful.
- Oral surgery: clipping tongue and/or the lingua frenum.
- Exorcisms and related faith healing rites.
- Hypnotism (mesmerism): postsuggestive states.
- Neurosurgery.
- Nutrition.
- Drugs.
- Chiropractics.
- Oral mechanistic manipulation drills.
- Autosuggestive techniques.

- Sociodrama.
- Desensitization methods
- Rote drill methods.
- Classical conditioning methods.
- Behavior modification methods.
- Biofeedback methods.
- Delayed auditory feedback methods.
- Relaxation and related bodily control methods.
- Acupuncture.
- Transcendental meditation and related guru techniques.
- Avoidance and/or distraction techniques.
- Psychotherapy/psychoanalytic methods.
- Mental-visualization methods.
- Assorted psychological approaches.
- Guidance/counseling methods.
- Self-help therapy methods.
- Auditory-masking devices.
- Voice-control masking devices.
- Neuropsychological approaches.

It seems apparent that the great majority of these constitute primarily neurophysiologically based therapy approaches, designed to treat stutterers' dysfluency symptoms directly. Other approaches attempt to do so indirectly by applying varying psychological methods. What may not be as apparent is that, whether or not by design, the primary objective of these neurophysiological and psychological approaches is their common attempts to separate the dysfluency behaviors from the stutterers.

This objective is obviously more practical than the medical approach, which endeavors to separate the patient from the disease. Unlike a disease, stuttering obviously cannot exist separate from the individual. As a result of the intimate interacting relationships of the individual's psychosocial experiences and his dysfluency behaviors, both are and should be treated as being one and the same.

Limitations of neurophysiologically based therapy approaches

There is a somewhat annoying consistency in the literature regarding its extensive reporting on research studies alluding to many forms of inherent or acquired, sensory, organic, neurological, neurotic, etc., behavioral symptoms and deficits to attribute to stuttering (as a cause or effect), and the predominantly neurophysiologically based approaches reported for treating stuttering.

This consistency is subject to question, because many of the conclusions relating to these symptoms and deficits, as well as the therapy approaches, consisted mainly of speculative generalizations. Yet, this would not justify concluding that any of these neurophysiologically based approaches are inadequate for treating stuttering. We may contend, however, for reasons stated above, that this consistency has contributed to the emphasis within training and clinic programs on the use of neurophysiologically based methods, which has led to the rigidity and limitations of current remedial approaches.

Proper research and their publications, particularly when sufficient knowledge is wanting, are needed and welcomed. If, however, the literature had reported only 20% of the widely diverse range of behavioral symptoms and deficits attributed to stuttering, Bloodstein would, no doubt, still have been of a mind, as quoted earlier, to question:

> Can the 'typical stutterer' be depicted to be: anally fixated, brain-damaged with atypical cortical dominance, inadequate of sound-mindedness; to possess inter-aural-phase disparities, lower auditory pain thresholds, vascular and biochemical imbalances, and/or a multiple of other differential anomalies?

Two basic problems relate to the treatment of stuttering. These are the frequency of the individual's repeated episodes of dysfluency behaviors, and the conditions that promote these repeated episodes. Advocates of neurophysiologically based therapy approaches, whether knowingly or not, generally assume that to treat mainly the individual's stuttering behaviors will serve to reduce the episodes and severity of these behaviors, and as a positive consequence, also his related psychosocial problems.

Comments: in spite of the hopeful logic of these advocates, these objectives nevertheless reflect the remedial limitations of current clinic programs in their dominant reliance on neurophysiologically based self-therapy methods. Consequently, self-therapy methods, rather than enhancing fluent speech may tend to reinforce the conditions that promote the individual's repeated episodes of stuttering behaviors.

Self-therapy techniques and limitations

> If all the king's horses, and all the king's men could not put Humpty-Dumpty together again, then, why not let Humpty-Dumpty try to put himself together again?

Clinic programs for the most part rely on mechanistic manipulation techniques, such as controls, starters, avoidances, conditioners, desensitization, distractors, relaxation measures, etc., as speech aids, to enable clients to gain ready availability of their developed speech fluency. Clinic programs generally advise against the use of coping adjustment methods, yet the techniques they more commonly employ tend to be 'the same horses of a difference color', i.e. self-therapy methods

The self-therapy techniques administered by clinic programs may, as a result of their designs, seem to aid fluent speech for longer periods than the somewhat impulsive coping methods stutterers employ on their own. The limitations of clinic techniques to obtain consistent beneficial results are, however, evident in the many clients, who have previously participated within one or more professional or pseudoprofessional programs. There is also the loss of confidence expressed by many, including a good number who, sustained by hope and need, continue to seek these programs.

> *Comments*: perhaps, there are some things particular to stuttering or stutterers, which tend to inhibit their dyfluency behaviors from responding consistently to self-therapy methods? Or could it be that self-therapy methods, and/or possibly how they are commonly administered, are counterproductive, in that they tend to promote the individuals repeated episodes of stuttering behaviors?

About 2300 years ago, Demosthenes, a famed Greek orator, administered self-therapy methods to control his stuttering behaviors. He used distraction (pebbles in his mouth) and masking (noise of the pounding surf) techniques to suppress them. Judging from his famed achievements as an orator, his self-administered therapy apparently met with good success.

Since Demosthenes' use of self-therapy methods, we have, after centuries of attacking stuttering with an awesome array of professional and pseudoprofessional approaches, apparently come full circle in the relatively recent emphasis on the use of self-therapy and masking feedback techniques, particularly with adult stutterers. Why, then, have past and current therapy programs using similar and more sophistocated techniques apparently failed consistently to gain comparable successful results?

Handbook: *Self-therapy for the Adult Stutterer*

None of the comments that follow intend any negative criticisms of the Speech Foundation's sponsorship of this handbook, or of its contributors. On the contrary, the Speech Foundation, and the contributing authors, are to be highly commended for their sincere concern and services on behalf of stutterers. We are rather objectively concerned with the limitations of self-therapy techniques and/or their methods of administration to obtain more beneficial and consistent therapy results.

The administration of self-therapy methods in the treatment of stuttering behaviors has been formalized within the Speech Foundation of America's sponsored handbook, *Self-therapy for the Adult Stutterer* (Fraser, 1988). This handbook offers, within its well-intentioned program for adult stutterers of heal thyself at home, a compendium of advice and recommended self-therapy techniques contributed by many leading authorities. According to the handbook, this program was designed to enable adult stutterers, for whom professional services are either unaffordable, unavailable or undesirable, to self-administer for their stuttering behaviors.

The handbook's self-therapy program appears to be highly elastic, giving the impression of an apparent one-size-for-all eclectic design to its approach. This would appear to be contrary to established concepts on individual human differences. Why emphasize the need for appropriate diagnostic and prognostic procedures, when all are apparently subject to the same therapy methods?

Stutterers might be authorities on their experiences as stutterers, but not necessarily with regard to the complexities relating to diagnosis and treatment of their dysfluency behaviors. It is, therefore, doubtful that the sole use of the handbook can provide sufficient, proper, professional, diagnostic, prognostic or therapy guidance, as well as the necessary motivational supports required.

The handbook's many recommended self-therapy procedures would tend to place excessive demands on the abilities of stutterers to self-administer for their differential stuttering behaviors without formal training. In this regard, we might ask:

> Why require speech therapists to undertake years of university training, with many hours of clinical practice, and earn clinical certifications to administer these methods, when, for stutterers, a handbook on self-therapy might apparently suffice?

In this regard, adult stutterers, who have attempted to participate in the handbook's program, complained of confusion, not only in assessing their stuttering behaviors, but also in determining which of the many methods recommended might meet their remedial needs best. One adult summed up these difficulties with the following comment:

> Trying to treat my stuttering from all the methods in the handbook, was like trying to learn to swim by taking a shower. There may be lots of water, but what can you do with it?

The motivation comments and self-therapy techniques contained within the the Speech Foundation's handbook were contributed by leading authorities on stuttering. Many of these contributors direct university and college programs for training speech and therapists, as well as clinic services for stutterers. Can we, therefore, assume that their recommended neurophysiological approaches for treating stuttering, evident in their motivating comments and self-therapy techniques, are similarly reflected in their training and clinic programs which, more or less, may be typical of most American training and clinic programs?

A particularly disturbing aspect of the handbook relates to the direct, and apparently uncompromising, assertions by its many contributors that the total responsibility for the successes of its self-therapy program rest entirely with the adult stutterers. The readers should reflect on the motivational context and tone of the following comments quoted directly from the handbook:

> The stutterer must conquer his own problems – no one else can do the job for you.
>
> Accept the fact that you have a serious problem. Stand squarely on both feet, place your shoulders back and begin earnestly to attack your problem.
>
> A valuable precondition for successful therapy is the deep inner conviction of the stutterer in the management of his disorder, combined with a fighting spirit and a readiness to undergo hardships and deprivation if needed. Hopelessness, pessimism and passivity being the deadliest foes to self-improvement.
>
> Don't ever forget that even if you went to the most knowledgeable expert in the country the correction of stuttering is a do-it-yourself project. Stuttering is your problem.
>
> The stutterer develops emotional reactions which permeate his soul, affect his will, and upset his mind.
>
> If you are like most of the million and one stutterers in this country, adequate clinical treatment will not be available to you. Whatever you do you will have to be pretty much on your own with what ideas and sources.
>
> Somehow you must learn to desensitize yourself to the reactions of others and refuse to let people's actual or imagined responses to your stuttering continue to affect your mental health or peace of mind.

Adult stutterers, reporting on their attempts to participate in this program, responded negatively to these comments. These comments were regarded to typify the 'go it alone experiences', often endured throughout their late teens and adult lives. Stutterers were burdened with such experiences, long before professional clinic programs became available. Would there have been the need for the large increase in clinic programs over the last 50 years, if stutterers had been consistently successful in self-administering their stuttering behaviors?

To place total responsibility for the administration and results of self-therapy on the stutterers, as many contributors to the handbook strongly asserted, would tend to foster preoccupations with means, outcomes, doubts, etc., which distracts from their objectives for participating in the program. Such distractions can disturb the stability of their readiness SETs to perform their developed speech. In addition, such preoccupations might also contribute to the diminishing value of the manipulation technique as speech aids.

Speech is a basic and most essential human tool. The young child's dependence on speech gratification experiences promoted his use and development of speech as a readily available means for communicating, and adjusting (coming to terms), with his various socioenvironments throughout his life. Self-therapy techniques which do not accord the adult stutterers consistent speech gratification experiences will not, therefore, promote stable readiness SETs, nor the positive neuropsychological conditions required for appreciably reducing, if not totally eliminating, his stuttering behavior.

Manipulation techniques, administered in self-therapy, generally consist of non-speech behavioral artifacts (referred to earlier), to enable the stutterer to effect fluent speech. In spite of the tendency of such artifacts to diminish as speech aids, the individual will persist in their usage as speech-related stuggles, to sustain even their limited value as speech aids. These struggles tend to foster the negative neuropsychological conditions, which promote them in becoming associated additions to the individual's repetoire of stuttering behaviors, formed within the secondary non-speech motor program.

The associated stuttering behaviors tend to reflect the extraneous movements of the particular coping manipulation techniques used, and often become the more pronounced and overtly obvious facial,

Comments: the above relates to the consistency of both the individual's developed speech and his non-speech stuttering behaviors. Fluent speech is not the problem, but rather the ready availability of its use, which is determined by the status of his readiness SETs and neuropsychological conditions. These factors effectively influence the activation of the motor programs relative to the neurophysiological motor processes for each: developed speech or stuttering behaviors.

This consistency is evident during his episodes of stuttering behaviors, which display disruptions to the forward flow of the automated neurophysiological motor processes for his developed speech with extraneous non-speech movements. This consistency strongly suggests the formation of each, as different automated neurophysiological motor processes, within different motor programs, fostered and activated by different neuropsychological conditions.

Considering the above, it would appear that to treat stutterers with more success would require more than self-therapy manipulation techniques. Such techniques may have a proper, yet limited place within the scope of a comprehensive therapy program. When, however, such techniques constitute the primary means for effecting control, avoidance, suppression, etc. of stuttering behaviors, the results are often the stilted robotization of stutterers' fluent speech performances.

head and bodily manifestations of the individual's stuttering behaviors. The individual's preoccupations with self-perceptions of these behaviors, and the perceptions of others, contribute to the traumatic neuropsychological conditions: feelings of helplessness, negative emotional responses, disturbed readiness SETs and negative anticipations, which promote his repeated episodes of stuttering behaviors.

The generally restrictive setting of clinic programs

A questionaire submitted to 200 university and college speech and hearing departments, during the early 1980s, surprisingly obtained 104 responses. One of the five questions asked was: 'To what extent does your clinic program for treating stutterers provide opportunities to use their clinic trainings within their daily lives?'

All but eleven reported assigning tasks requiring teenage and adult clients to visit or telephone local stores, public offices, etc., or to approach strangers, to express certain requests. These tasks are discussed during clinic sessions to enable clients to gain insights from these experiences. Eighty-nine reported family counseling, and 22 provided social meetings for clients and family members, from one to two evenings per month. Twenty-four were referred to annual workshops administered by guest authorities on stuttering. Two reported two-week summer camp workshops for young stutterers.

These responses were assumed to be somewhat typical of clinic programs nation-wide, with regard to limiting the scope of their therapy methods mainly to within the confines of their clinic environments. This suggested that the therapy procedures administered by these, and most clinic programs, adhered primarily to subjecting clients with mechanistic manipulation techniques, by which they might self-administer to their speech needs within their daily experiences.

Mechanistic manipulation techniques to control, suppress, avoid, etc., stuttering behaviors, whether or not designed, are measures intended to separate the clients from their stuttering behaviors. Stutterers do not, however, leave their psychosocial problems in limbo outside therapy rooms while being subjected to mechanistic manipulative programming for fluent speech. To fail to account for the effective influences of the client's psychosocial problems while attempting to treat his stuttering behaviors is analogous to attempting to treat the aggravating bee stings, while ignoring the continued attacks of the bees.

Clinic programs often succeed, within their artificial speech environments, to demonstate clients' ability to perform fluent speech. Attempts to motivate transference of these fluent speech performances to within the client's daily environments often, however, do not succeed. This may well result from the absence of significant changes in disturbing conditions within the clients' real life environments, which contribute to sustainment of their stuttering behaviors. Failure to implement appropriate measures to effect realistic transference of the improvements obtained might also relate to notions that such transference is a major responsibility of the clients.

Clinic programs, as reported above, attempt to provide real life speech experiences by assigning clients such tasks as visiting or telephoning local stores, public offices, etc., or talking to strangers. These, however, are artificial speech events, as are the social evenings, which also lack the sudden urgencies for readily available speech more common to the realities of clients' daily experiences as stutterers.

Furthermore, the clients seemingly improved fluent speech performances might result mainly from their temporary adaptations to the artificial, non-stressful clinic environments, rather than to the therapy techniques applied. The negative neuropsychological conditions that evoke their episodes of stuttering behaviors are not being dealt with. On the contrary, they remain unchanged, waiting outside the clinic to impose their frustrating influences on clients' speech efforts.

In summary: the limitations of current clinic programs, as with past programs, center on their tendency to attempt to treat the behavior symptoms of stuttering more directly than the clients themselves. In addition, they attempt to do so within the artificial, relatively meaningless and unrealistic confines of their clinic setting. In spite of the therapy methods employed within the clinic, this continues to leave the clients vunerable to the negative psychosocial experiences, which promote the conditions for their repeated episodes of stuttering behaviors.

Comments: the clinic's apparent lack of programs for providing experiences related to their clients' real life needs tends to be somewhat alien to our advanced concepts of learning about and shaping human behaviors. Failure to do so deprives them of the necessary motivation to sustain their use of self-therapy techniques learned within the clinic, and transference of the probable results. To impose the total responsibilities for the successs of their self-therapy efforts on them is counterproductive. Whether these negative factors are the result of a lack of understanding or concern, or of rigid adherence to traditional procedures, is difficult to ascertain.

The above references to the limitations deemed to be typical of clinic programs are presented in the manner of an umpire officiating a sports event. The methods are judged, as they are believed to be seen, without criticism of the competence of the personnel.

Inadvertent tendency of clinic programs to reflect public attitudes towards stutterers

Is it possible that the limitations, expressed above, which apparently contribute to the restrictions of clinic programs in their provision of consistent beneficial therapy, might relate somehow to long-held public attitudes towards stutterers? The expression of such attitudes may, over the years, have become more subtle, but nevertheless effective, particularly with regard to the problems of adult stutterers, which are still considered to be more a matter of personal rather than public concern.

Until the last 120 years or so, most Western societies were primarily farming cultures; thus, work ability valued manual rather than speech skills. Stutterers were not generally disadvantaged from pursuing farming or other basically manual trades. In spite of certain social stigmas fostered mostly by ignorance, whatever problems might relate to their manner of speaking were regarded as mainly personal,

With the growth of cities, however, vocations relating to industry, mercantile trades, public services, education, law, medicine, etc., placed ever-increasing demands on speech skills. Societies grow and survive by maintaining standards deemed to promote the common good, stability and progress. Societies do not, however, always provide an equal distribution of the common good, stability or progress to all its members, particularly to those regarded as atypical or limited in their potential to contribute to the common good.

This rapid expansion of industry, business and other professional fields provided opportunities previously available only to relatively small élite sections of society. These expanded opportunities placed increased emphasis on communication (speech) skills. When good speech therefore became equated with competence, stutterers became work liabilities.

The general public tends to be slow in its awareness and acknowledgment of those of its members who become disadvantaged by being regarded as limited in their potential to meet standards of competence for professional and business skills. Consequently, although the increased public demands for speech skills tended to draw increased attention to stutterers, there was no comparable interest drawn towards regarding their problems as ones of public concern.

With the greater attention and need for communication skills, university and colleges expanded their training programs to include speech and hearing departments. Starting in the late 1940s, extended interest in research on stuttering appeared to parallel the pursuit of degrees. Over the following years, there was a proliferation of research designed to break the etiological puzzle of stuttering. The apparent difficulties led to a less mysterious and more bountiful search for organic and functional symptoms and deficits that might be attributable to stuttering and stutterers.

Popular publications and professional journals seemed to be in competition to enlighten the public about stuttering. Popular publications, in particular, used tentative research studies to support pseudo-professional and misleading claims relating to causes, symptoms, prevention and/or treatment of stuttering. How is the public to think and act towards stutterers, when its professional members appear to support misconceptions of stuttering and misrepresentations of stutterers?

Some years ago, a popular John Wayne movie depicted a young cowhand being treated harshly for stuttering, because he should act like a man and could stop stuttering if he really tried. What impressions did this have on public attitudes towards stutterers, and upon stutterers? Although not inferring any causal relationship with the above movie, we could ponder:

> Could not the strong assertions, by the contributors to the handbook on self-therapy, obligating stutterers to total responsibility, inadvertently reflect the attitude shown towards the young stutterer in the above movie?

There was also a general tendency to expect stutterers to pursue interests and vocations that place minimum demands on speech skills for attaining some degree of success. Stutterers are often counselled to cope with their problems, by compromising their talents, interests and vocational aspirations. Although this might appear to be in their best interest, years of working with professional and other public groups, on behalf of stutterers, have led me to regard such compromise as disadvantaging stutterers – by their own consent.

> *Comments*: the 'It is your total responsibility' and the 'You must go it alone' attitudes towards adult stutterers are also implied in the somewhat contradictory tendency of clinic programs to attempt to treat clients' stuttering behaviors, while stressing their need to adjust to being stutterers. Why is there this need to allude to limitations, if not possible failure, when positive anticipations contribute to success? What doubts are being touched upon, and possibly misplaced?

Psychosocial bases for treating stutterers: responsibilities, motivations and opportunities

Responsibilities

Webster's Dictionary defines responsibility as:

A thing or person for whom one is responsible.

Clinic programs might inadvertently not be fulfilling their total responsibility, or aware of the extent of their need to do so. This observation tends to be supported by the comments of many of the contributors to the handbook *Self-therapy for the Adult Stutterer* (Fraser, 1988), which strongly assert that the total responsibility for the success of their proposed self-therapy program rests squarely on the stutterers. As authorities on stuttering, are their assertions typical of their own program and clinic programs in general?

Furthermore, it would seem reasonable to contend that it is within the context of the clinics' total responsibility not only to be aware of the limitations of their programs, but also to seek practical and effective means for reducing the restrictions imposed on their remedial objectives by such limitations. Yet, clinic programs seem to be frozen to adherence to traditional methods, which center on treating stuttering behaviors within relatively sterile confines, in a manner that is rather like providing Band-aid therapy.

Stuttering behaviors do not form, or repeatedly occur, within a social vacuum. On the contrary, these behaviors occur within real life situations, resulting from the disturbing conditions caused by a breakdown in the on-going interactions between the individual and his socioenvironment. It would seem a necessary responsibility of clinic programs to attempt to make a proper determination of the effects of these conditions on their clients' potential to cooperate, as well as their benefit from participation in their programs.

It is, therefore, suggested that clinic programs might endeavor to help repair this breakdown. They might do so by seeking means to extend the responsibility of their programs *beyond the confines* of their relatively artificial environments. By better understanding of a client's real world of frustrated needs and experiences, they might undertake approaches that can help effectively to reduce the traumatic neuropsychological conditions which promote and activate that client's repeated episodes of stuttering behaviors.

By assuming a more equitable and active share of their total responsibility, clinic programs can help towards relieving clients of the 'You must go-it-alone experiences'. The negative emotional responses of clients' preoccupations with such experiences can contribute to the instability of their readiness SETs for speech, which can effectively hamper their motivations and potentials to participate fully and benefit from therapy.

In summary: most current clinic programs continue to rely, in spite of acknowledged limitations, mainly on traditional mechanistic/manipulative techniques, applied within relatively artificial contexts, for controlling, avoiding, suppressing, eliminating, etc., stuttering behaviors. Although these techniques may or may not be spiced with varying psychological methods, they nevertheless attempt to deal more with the stuttering behaviors than with the conditions that promote these behaviors.

Comments: restrictive therapy results, as stated above, will tend to continue until clinic programs extend their therapy responsibilities to consider the conditions that disrupt their clients' efforts to use their developed speech as a readily available means to achieve their needs and desired objectives. It is after all within these external conditions that clients are subjected to the direct and indirect consequences of the negative psychosocial factors, which contribute to sustaining their repeated episodes of stuttering behaviors.

The above suggests the need of clinic programs to more equitably share in the provision of appropriate socially based supports for obtaining the best possible remedial results. Without implementation of mutually clarified responsibilities, most therapy approaches may continue to prove counterproductive not only to the therapy results of such programs, but also to the realistic needs of the clients.

The readers might note a certain critical, and perhaps polemic, tone to the above reference to the status responsibilities of clinic programs. This is most certainly not intended to denigrate the competence of the highly valued and ethical efforts of clinic programs to treat their clients. This tone could better reflect the eagerness, and perhaps urgency, of the author's belief that there may well be more realistic and beneficially productive therapy approaches for treating the problems common to stuttering.

Motivations

Success is the product of succeeding.

Piaget regarded speech as a primary motivational power by which the child learned skills from which they benefited. Speech, however, is also a basic tool developed primarily by the on-going motivations (gratifications) its use provides. It would seem, therefore, that, for stutterers to attempt to learn to change their speech performances, mainly to benefit from its change, would tend to detract from its effectiveness as a motivational power for treating the basic problems of stuttering.

Furthermore, to attempt to change one's speech performance requires perceptions and preoccupations with motives, methods and available or potential opportunites from which one might benefit. Changes in speech are thus perceived as necessary means towards obtaining perceptions of anticipated gratifications. Such preoccupations, on the contrary, tend to work against the objectives of therapy methods applied. Stutterers do not require learning of what they already have, namely developed speech. What they do require are practical motivations, which can promote the ready availability of their developed speech.

If the desire for fluent speech alone was sufficient motivation for stutterers to use the self-therapy techniques within their daily socio-environments, it would still be doubful that consistent beneficial results would be obtained. Nor have consistent results been obtained, when their desires for fluent speech have been supported by participation in traditional clinic programs. Instead, as a result of their initial successess with manipulative techniques, some clients form a certain dependence on them, This has tended to make them susceptible to exploitation by pseudoprofessional programs, promising cures at costs they can ill afford.

A necessary motivating criterion for the success of therapy methods would require both the clients and the program administrators to have mutual understanding of the basic objectives of the methods to be applied. Ethical clinic programs foster therapy objectives that are deemed to be realistic, practical and in the best interests of their clients. Clinics can, however, only offer tentative objectives and results, whereas clients tend to harbor expectations for total cures. Unless such differences in objectives are properly clarified, clients' motivations, and thus their efforts to participate fully in the therapy program, can be negatively affected.

The influence of these differences seems to be evident in the form of subjective aggressive–passive attitudes that stutterers have exhibited in the apparent inconsistencies in the results of their efforts to self-administer therapy techniques. These attitudes tend to be noted more in stutterers who have been subjected to previously unsuccessful therapy experiences. These differences may also relate to the stubborn resistance stuttering behaviors have long shown towards a multiplicity of past and current remedial approaches.

It would seem that the clients should be sufficiently motivated by the apparent improvements in speech fluency, experienced within the clinic setting, to self-administer the techniques applied more consistently, within their socioenvironments, to sustain these results. Yet, their motivations to do so often tend to be frustrated by the limited, and diminishing, value provided by speech aid techniques for effecting fluent speech outside the clinic setting.

Comments: it would seem evident that, for stutterers to engage in therapy, while subject to the external socioenvironmental conditions that tend to disadvantage them, can serve to restrict, or negate, the possible successes of their therapy efforts. There would therefore appear to be an apparent need for clinic programs that direct proper attention to those external conditions that tend to inhibit their clients' motivations, and thus, the results of their participation in the programs.

Opportunities: essential factors in treating stuttering

In previous chapters, I have endeavored to present a background in support of the following main contentions:

1. Stuttering, in spite of exhibiting disordered speech, cannot properly be regarded as a speech disorder and, thus, cannot be treated by standard manipulation speech or related therapy methods, which commonly require considerable preoccupation with the applied methods to effect correction.

   Correction of fluent speech is not a problem in relation to stuttering behaviors, because such behaviors do not inhibit children's development of the neurophysiological motor processes for fluent speech. Nor do they alter these developed motor speech processes on their formation.

   Furthermore, for the stutterer, undue preoccupation with the techniques applied can have negative consequences on the therapy results. Also, the disruptive non-speech dysfluency behaviors cannot be treated separately from the conditions that promote and activate their repeated occurrences.
2. Requiring that clients accept sole responsibility for the results of their participation in clinic programs tends to compound the psychosocial conditions that disadvantaged them from opportunities to pursue their interests and desired vocations in the first place. Also, this can inhibit their motivation and thus their potential to benefit from therapy.
3. Restricting therapy programs to the clinic environment cannot properly account for the disturbing psychosocial influences that tend to promote clients' traumatic neuropsychological conditions, and activate their repeated episodes of stuttering behaviors. Nor do they promote the necessary transference of clients' seemingly improved speech fluency to his outside environment.
4. The primary reliance of clinic programs on the application of mechanistic manipulation techniques, to treat mainly their clients' stuttering behaviors, tends to produce inconsistent therapy results. The efforts of the clients to self-administer these techniques can also contribute towards the conditions that promote their repeated episodes of these disruptive behaviors.
5. A major limitation of therapy program, which relies mainly on its manipulation techniques, is evident in failure to provide sufficient motivational supports for the therapy approaches.
6. The stutterer's preoccupations with his uncertain dependence on speech leads to negative emotional responses to disturbing percep-

tions of external stimuli (conditions), and negative anticipations, which evoke traumatic neuropsychologial conditions, manifesting reactions as episodes of stuttering behaviors, which disrupt the forward flow of his developed speech.

7. Therapy for stutterers requires approaches that endeavor to treat the disturbing psychosocial conditions, related to the breakdown in the interactions between the stutterers and their socioenvironments. As a consequence of this breakdown, the availability of their developed speech is subject to disruptive episodes of non-speech dysfluency behaviors, activated by traumatic neuropsychological conditions, and evoked by negative perceptions and emotional responses to external speech-related stimuli.

In consideration of the above and preceding discussions, it seems that:

1. The primary means for providing therapy programs for treating stutterers should center on efforts to repair the breakdown in their interactions with socioenvironments. This will serve towards reducing the traumatic neuropsychological conditions that promote and activate the episodes of dysfluency behaviors, disrupting the forward flow of their developed speech.
2. The primary objective of therapy programs should enable stutterers to gain the ready availability of their developed speech, rather than employ techniques directly on their stuttering behaviors.

To provide both the above primary means and objective, it is further suggested that clinic programs should extend the responsibility of their therapy programs beyond the artificial confines of the clinic setting. By doing so, clinic programs can better understand and treat more directly the disturbing psychosocial conditions particular to each client, rather than attempt to work directly on their stuttering behaviors.

The primary means by which clinic programs can obtain the above primary objective is to deal directly with clients' disturbing psycho-social conditions. This involves actively assisting in seeking opportunities that can provide immediate and meaningful motivating speech gratification experiences related to clients' talents and vocational interests.

Within the design of such programs, clients can experience speech gratifications directly from the success of their participation in these opportunities. For stutterers to participate successfully in opportunities that accord immediate and consistent speech gratification experiences serves to motivate and reinforce the ready availability of their developed speech.

Understandably, stutterers must bear responsibility for their participation in clinic programs. Stutterers do not expect, demand or desire to be spoon-fed at the public trough. They do, however, need professional and public assistance within their therapy programs, which can help to accord them opportunities to experience speech gratification from success obtained in real life situations related to their interests and talents.

In summary: motivation is a complex neuropsychological stimulus, which can move a person to act consistently to effect desired changes in his performances of skills and/or behaviors. The most effective and reinforcing motivators should provide stutterers with opportunities for immediate and consistent speech gratification experiences, from the success of participation in meaningful and desired opportunities to succeed.

> *Comments*: the application of coping manipulation techniques, without appropriate professional and public assistance, will continue to subject stutterers to the tasks of attempting to administer self-therapy to a complex psychosocial behavior disorder, and use of limited effective techniques within relatively indifferent socioenvironments. To attempt successful therapy under such conditions might appear to be tantamount to attempting brain surgery with a meat cleaver.

Masking feedback devices

There are many techniques and devices that claim to provide stutterers with immediate fluent speech experiences. There are various glossopharyngeal and laryngeal coping adjustment techniques, including the Valsalva hypothesis, which claim to give immediate fluent speech experiences by relieving phonatory and/or speech breath blocks. Research relating to the validity of most of these techniques and devices is still wanting.

Whether such basically self-therapy techniques can consistently produce fluent speech experiences is relative only to the final results; without proper meaningful support these would tend, like manipulation techniques, to diminish in value as a speech aid. There are also various types of artificial electro-device which claim to provide immediate fluent speech experience. Some of the more prominent of these are discussed below.

Demosthenes accompanied his use of pebbles with the masking effects of the surf pounding against the shore to support his self-therapy efforts to treat his stuttering behaviors. His continued use of these distraction techniques does not alter the contention that his motivations for doing so were fostered mainly by the immediate speech successes experienced, without the need to be preoccupied with self-administration of these distraction techniques. It was this notion of his self-therapy efforts that, many years ago, influenced my approach to treating stutterers themselves rather than their dysfluency behaviors. It would appear, in this regard, that Demosthenes was many centuries ahead of his time.

The use of masking feedback devices with stutterers is not a new innovation. Its use with stutterers had, however, been limited as well as being subject to professional controversy (Ryan, 1979). Considerable advancement in construction and performances has, however, greatly improved their dependability as a complementary therapy aid for enhancing stutterers' performance of fluent speech.

Masking feedback devices have been used mainly within clinic programs, in conjunction with standard therapy methods, to enable stutterers to experience relatively immediate fluent speech. Such experiences were intended to enable clients to self-visualize the movements of their oral and vocal mechanisms in their basic use of self-control/manipulation methods to effect fluent speech.

These devices are still considered of value for training stutterers in self-visualization of fluent speech functions. The more current use of these devices is, however, intended to avoid the considerably longer time, and less certain results, required for learning to self-administer the more standard manipulation or desensitization techniques for controlling, suppressing, avoiding, etc., stuttering behaviors.

The handbook on self-therapy advised against the use of artificial devices to augment self-therapy, in case the user became overly dependent on them. Dependence is, however, relative to the value of the needs served. Do we question the common dependence on wearing glasses or using hearing aids to aid sensory deficits? We live within a highly technotronic society, which has produced remarkable devices for restoring severely disturbed sensory and motor functions, as well as for sustaining life.

Artificial devices, such as the electro-larynx, and palatal and dental prostheses, are commonly used for restoring or improving speech functions. Early experiences with delayed auditory feedback devices found that they provided more immediate fluent speech experiences than manipulation techniques. There were, however, obvious inconsistencies in clients' retention of fluent speech without use of the devices, particularly outside the clinic setting.

In later work, particularly with stutterers in their late teens or adults, no manipulation techniques were applied or allowed. It had become increasingly apparent that the use of auditory masking and masking feedback devices, in conjunction with a program centered on treating stutterers directly, rather than their dysfluency behaviors, obtains much quicker and more consistent and beneficial results. It was reasoned that providing fluent speech experiences alone, with the use of the devices, was not enough to promote the necessary reinforcements for enhancing consistency in their fluent speech performances, particularly without the use of the devices within their socioenvironments.

To promote the necessary reinforcements, the program implemented for working with the stutterers, rather than on their dysfluency behaviors, was designed to:

1. Avoid all need for the clients to be distracted by undue preoccupations with methods employed for the provision of fluent speech experiences. Proper adjustment and practice in the use of the devices served this objective.
2. Assist clients in obtaining needed opportunities that could provide them with immediate and consistent speech gratification experiences from success gained through participation in meaningful activities related to their interests and talents. This was intended to reinforce clients' dependence on speech as a readily available tool for obtaining gratification, rather than on preoccupation with fluent speech performance.

The movements for performing speech develop primarily as automated neurophysiological processes, which generally require no preoccupation with production for use as a readily available tool. A primary objective was to regain this natural function of speech.

To implement this program, it was necessary to extend the clinic program to the clients' socioenvironments, and assist them in acquiring desired opportunities, related to their needs and/or interests. Particular efforts were made to get the opportunities that clients had regarded they were disadvantaged from as a result of their stuttering, or were beyond the potentials of their speech. (Examples of these are depicted later in this chapter.)

> *Comments*: the use of these devices to provide clients with immediate speech fluency experiences offered an unexpected advantage, which was often used to good effect, in our efforts to provide meaningful opportunties. These devices, often surprisingly, enabled clients to demonstrate their ability to speak with fluency. This served towards altering their misunderstanding of and biased attitudes towards stuttering, which promoted their more ready cooperation.

The Edinburgh Masker

The Edinburgh Masker provides a masking tone activated by the speaker's voice. The speaker's voice is picked up by a throat microphone and transmitted to small receivers placed in the ears. The masking tone can be heard only by the speaker, and may be altered by variations in his voice productions. The rationale for the use of this device as quoted in the instructions is as follows:

> If the user, due to the masking effects of variable low frequency noise backgrounds, cannot hear himself stutter he will not be subjected to the disturbing influences of his stuttering behaviors.

The Edinburgh Masker is generally recommended primarily for mild to moderate adult stutterers, for whom it permits relatively immediate functional use of their developed fluent speech. Its use is regarded as avoiding the need for stutterers to undergo the more extensive and costly training common to traditional clinic programs. Also, the user is less likely to apply uncertain coping adjustment methods, which tend to become speech-related stuggles.

The Vocal Feedback Device

The Vocal Feedback Device (VFD), developed by Dr George Shames, works on the principle of vibrotactile feedback, which is intended to form a communication loop between the speaker's mind and his body. This communication loop is designed to allow the speaker, as its designer contends, to focus his mind firmly on the tasks necessary for production of clearly articulated speech.

This device uses a microphone and amplifier attached to a neck vibrator set within a sort of choker. As the user speaks, movements of his vocal folds are amplified and transmitted back through the choker. The user's sensitivity to the vibrations heightens awareness of his speech patterns so enhancing increased concentration. The speaker is thus reported to learn to control the tension and movements of his vocal folds as needed for fluent speech.

There are basic differences with regard to the form of feedback stimuli used by each of the Edinburgh and the VFD masking devices:

1. The Edinburgh Masker uses auditory feedback, whereas the VFD device relies on vibratory tactile (proprioceptive) feedback.
2. The Edinburgh Masker is regarded as requiring a minimum clinical training. The VFD device requires professionally guided clinical training in slow, careful speaking and desensitization therapy to obtain precise fluency shaping.
3. The Edinburgh Masker tends to require 'on and off' usage for an indefinite period. The VFD device endeavors to wean the client away from its use.

Delayed auditory feedback devices

These devices are based on the concept that, when the user talks into a microphone, his voice, heard through a headset, will be delayed by adjustable fractions of a second. The speaker would not thus be subject to distracting influences of his stuttering behaviors.

There are several versions of devices using delayed auditory feedback methods. One of the more recent was designed by David Kehoe. This device is essentially a DAF telephone for stutterers, which connects to the AT&T 700 series of telephones, and has an 'off-phone mode' for practice or face-to-face conversations. It consists of a Walkman-style headset with a built-in microphone and a Walkman-sized speech processor.

Perkins (1978) reported on the Kehoe DAF device as follows:

> We tested it in comparison with time-out, airflow, and other frequently used techniques and discovered that it had the most universal effect of establishing fluency promptly. Unlike the alternatives, it produces all but instant fluency regardless of severity, age or sex.

Practical applications of masking feedback devices

Experiences with earlier versions of DAF, and later the Edinburgh Maskers, with teenage and adult stutterers showed more readily available fluent speech, within relatively short periods, than did standard approaches. It is important to note that, until our program was extended beyond the confines of our clinic setting, attempts to treat clients' speech needs and objectives obtained mainly tentative results.

The use of these devises provided a particularly important psychological basis upon which to implement our program. Upon admission, extensive discussions were held with each client. Among the topics discussed was the nature of stuttering as a disruption to the availability of their developed speech, rather than as a speech disorder. Thus, the primary objective of the program was not to provide speech therapy, because none was needed, but rather to support this natural availability. This was relatively easy to demonstrate with the more immediate fluent speech experiences provided by use of the device. This also apparently relieved them of doubts relating to mastering the anticipated required techniques, which enhanced motivation.

Clients with moderate, as well as moderately severe, stuttering behaviors showed significant positive speech responses within relatively short periods. The efforts of our clinic to help towards the provision of increased opportunities for speech gratification experiences clearly supported their fluent speech experiences, with use of the devices. This was noted in their greater confidence and self-visualization for participation in speech events and served to stabilize their readiness

SETs for speech, which, in turn, reduced episodes of disturbing activation of their stuttering behaviors.

There were also definite indications of reduced tendency to exhibit disturbing psychosocial behaviors, such as negative anticipations, passivity, feelings of helplessness, avoidance, repressed anxieties and related emotional states. Reduction in these behaviors appeared to be reinforced with clients increasing their successful fluent speech experiences without the use of their devices.

Severe adult stutterers also derived notable gains in fluent speech experiences and yet required longer and greater effort than with less severe stutterers, as a result of initial reluctance and/or seeming inability to cooperate. They showed dependence on the devices and resistance to be weaned from using them. They came to regard the devices as something like spectacles or hearing aids.

In spite of their obvious dependence on the devices, these adults showed positive changes in assertiveness and self-confidence in their speech performances. These changes reflected greater self-visualization and positive anticipation of a more consistent performance of fluent speech. What was important to them was the greater consistency, even if limited, in their successful experiences within meaningful opportunities to obtain speech gratification experiences, long denied them because of their severe stuttering behaviors.

My experiences with the VFD and the Kehoe DAF are limited mainly to observation, reading of the literature and discussions with colleagues. Most of the literature and comments relating to effectiveness of these devices to provide immediate fluent speech experiences has, however, been favorable. I would therefore, in principle, favor their use within appropriate supportive programs as referred to above.

Comments: the main point is not, however, whether the use of this or that device can promote fluent speech experiences, but whether through their sole use fluent speech can be consistently effected, without the need to consider the negative psychosocial bases for stutterers' traumatic neuropsychological reactions. These reactions, we noted, tend to promote not only their repeated episodes of stuttering behaviors, but also the resistance of such behaviors to therapy methods.

Clinical reports

The following client reports are given only as examples, rather than as testimonials, of the beneficial and consistent results that can be typically obtained with stutterers. One of the most effective means for obtaining these results related directly to the supportive opportunities that provided more favorable conditions for reducing the effective negative influences of their respective psychosocial conditions. Another important factor was their increased self-confidence which, in part, related to their awareness of the sense of shared responsibities.

Although the reports refer to the use of artificial devices in conjunction with meaningful opportunities used by the therapy approaches, there were frequent occasions, particularly during the earlier years, when beneficial therapy successes were obtained without these devices. A main advantage of these devices is in an appreciable shortening of the time required to obtain favorable therapy results with moderate to moderately severe stutterers.

Case A

Janet, a 16-year-old, pleasantly attractive, shy appearing, high school student, exhibited moderate classical stuttering behaviors with obvious associated spasmodic clonic-like movements, mainly of her head, eyes and lips. She had participated in public school speech therapy programs on two occasions, and once in a private program, at the age of 9, 11 and 13 years, respectively.

Janet expressed interest in nursing, but stated that she had been advised to consider a more practical vocation. She had been teased by peers during her later elementary classes, but less since entering high school. Janet's parents, as well as her teachers, considered her to be 'kind of withdrawn from participating in social and class activities'.

Her current interest was to be a cheerleader, 'because they seem to have all the friends; besides it's something I can do well'. Janet had trained in a summer training camp for cheerleaders on two occasions. Believing herself to be qualified, and urged by her mother, she applied for a place on the team, but was not accepted. She felt that serious considerations were not granted to her because of her stuttering behaviors.

Janet showed reluctance to enter our program. She regarded her previous therapy to be 'a waste of time'. The objectives of our program, including its shared responsibility aspects and the functions of the DAF device, were discussed with Janet and her parents, who assured their full cooperation.

A trial session was arranged, during which Janet experienced the DAF device. Although still seeming reluctant, she agreed to three sessions per week. A week of orientation comprised discussions relating to her interests, attitudes and related feelings, and practice with the device. There were discussions about the nature of stuttering as a disruption to the availability of her developed speech, rather than as a speech disorder. The device was used to support these discussions, and to enhance motivation by providing relatively immediate better fluent speech experiences.

With her approval, contact was made with her gym teachers, who contended that Janet was denied a trial in the cheerleading team to avoid her embarrassment, and possible resentment by other members of the team. We discussed the fairness of Janet being disadvantaged for the convenience of others, and the benefits, in both speech and self-confidence, she might derive from the experiences as a cheerleader.

Permission was given to discuss Janet's interests and needs with the team members. It was agreed to grant her a trial, to see, as one member stated '. . . what she's got'. During a visit to her home, Janet displayed her cheerleading skills, which led to her being allowed to practice with the team on a trial basis. During some of the early clinic sessions, Janet, among other things, performed her cheerleading routines with the use of the device before several classes of student therapists, which included explaining her routines.

By the third week, following favorable discussions with her teachers, Janet was asked to wear the device in her classes. She could choose the classes, and had the option to participate orally as she might desire. These experiences were discussed in the sessions with emphasis on gratifying descriptions of her feelings and attitudes relating to her experiences. Changes in her attitude reflected reinforcement of self-confidence.

Janet was reported to be 'fitting in well' with the cheerleading routines, and with the team members. She was regarded to be ready to perform at the next weekly football game, and did quite well. Although she used the device during practice sessions, she reported not using it during the game, because the background noise within the stadium provided effective masking support. She did well on her initial debut, and at later sports events, without relying on the DAF device. She felt accepted as a member of the team.

Janet reported that her classroom teachers were pleasantly surprised with her improved participation in class activities. During these detailed discussions of her classroom experiences, attention was centered mainly on their positive aspects. She showed good insight and growing self-confidence in these experiences. With her teachers' approval, she was asked to consider explaining her use of the device and cheerleading routines before her classes.

By the fourth week, Janet's parents provided her with her own DAF device. They reported evident positive changes in her attitudes and social activities, with apparent growth in self-confidence, and in the quality of her speech performances. She added ornaments to the handband of the device and cheerleading which gave it a decorative appearance.

By the sixth week, she was wearing the device less at home, at the clinic and in some of her classes. Although pleased with her progress, she attributed the success of her improved speech experiences to the support and the opportunities others had provided. She was told to be proud of her own efforts, because opportunities are the doors she had to enter by herself.

During week eight, Janet did not rely on the device during her clinic sessions. She relied on it mainly while shopping, when visiting relatives or friends, and in those classes which she regarded as still somewhat uncertain, more because of difficulty with the course content than because of her reluctance to participate orally.

After the tenth week, it was considered prudent to release Janet, with her approval, from her clinic sessions which, by the end of the sixth week, had been reduced to one session per week. There was very noticeable and consistent reduction in her stuttering behaviors, and particularly the moderate associated (facial bodily) behaviors. She was, however, invited to visit the clinic as she might either feel necessary or desire.

Follow-up reports showed Janet's continued progress in self-confidence and positive anticipation towards participating within her classes and other social activities. Her speech gratification experiences relate to meaningful real life needs and aspirations. She reported her decision to give serious consideration to pursuing her interests in a nursing career, and arranged an interview with the head nurse at the local hospital.

Two years later, Janet visited the clinic to inform us of her enrollment in a pre-nursing university program. She reported and showed significant stability in her fluent speech performances, as well as confidence in the ready availability of her speech, particularly within situations formerly deemed uncomfortable. She commented on her occasional use of her DAF device within particular situations mainly for sustaining her self-confidence.

Case B

Marvin, a 20-year-old, tall, well-built young man, exhibited moderate classical stuttering behaviors, with clonic–labial and glottal blockages. There were also associated tic-like facial head movements, with some mild extraneous associated bodily movements.

Marvin was brought to the university clinic by his father, who was quite insistent on speaking for him. His father reported that Marvin, as a result of his stuttering behaviors, had been taunted during his earlier school years, and was, because of his size, inclined to show hostility and self-consciousnes. He stated that Marvin was very interested in geology, but lacked the confidence to pursue his interest at university level.

Marvin had attended two public school speech programs between the ages of 8 and 13 years. His father contended that these programs '. . . did not seem to help, but that,' . . .perhaps, he may not have done his best'. Marvin, however, later claimed that he did not understand what was being attempted or expected of him in these programs. He stated, 'Mostly I had to read from children's books and repeat words I stuttterered over and over'.

The father was requested to leave to allow private discussion with Marvin, who seemed reluctant to be in the clinic. Marvin, however, did confirm his interests in geology, as well as the desire to pursue university training. His fears to do so centered on his stuttering, which he regarded would be a problem not only within his classes, but also as a source of personal and social problems away from home.

Marvin had twice deferred application for admission to the university. His father had strongly urged him to enroll in the coming fall semester, with depictions of a bleak and unhappy future should he fail to enroll. The program and its objectives were explained, including the functions of the Edinburgh Masker. Marvin at first appeared to be somewhat doubtful with regard to the potentials of the masker to assist him in producing fluent speech more easily. He also seemed reluctant to '. . . having to wearing a gadget around my throat all the time'. After some recorded trials with the device were re-played, he did express interest by asking what would be required.

Marvin's interest in geology appeared to be well supported by his evident knowledge of fossils found in various areas of the world, which he apparently enjoyed describing. When it was suggested that his interests in geology might have been motivated by primarily physical activities, rather than speech demands, he shrugged and stated, 'Perhaps, but I really like it'.

With his father present, the program and objectives were explained once more. A one-week trial period of three sessions was agreed upon, with the option to continue left entirely to Marvin. It was advised that he attend these sessions alone, which required that he drive about 35 miles from his home, to which he quickly agreed.

During this trial week with the masker, we discussed Marvin's interests, primary objectives and self-images. He stated that his main objective was: 'To speak anywhere, easily without stuttering.' He acknowledged his tendency to hostility when taunted about his stuttering, or when frustrated by difficulties in communicating. He responded well to the device, and was quite pleased to experience immediate reduction in his stuttering behaviors. He agreed to continue in the program.

By week 3, Marvin was permitted to use the device outside the clinic. His confidence in the use of device increased. With his approval and use of the masker, it was arranged for him to discuss his interest in geology with members of the university geology department. He reported that these discussions went better than he had expected and stated that he had been invited to sit in on two of the geology classes, and to go on two of their weekend field trips. He reported on each visit, and on his enjoyment of these experiences.

At the start of the fall semester, his parents presented Marvin with an Edinburgh Masker, which he used in his classes. His teachers were very cooperative. He stated that he was participating more in the classroom. It was evident that he enjoyed detailing the discussions he had with classmates. During his clinic sessions, in spite of wearing the device, he relied on its use less frequently. He further assured that he would also attempt to do so during his classes, at home and in other speech situations. Visiting his home, his parents expressed satisfaction with Martin's speech progress, his general attitudes and social behaviors.

By week 8, Marvin's clinic sessions were reduced to one per week. Three weeks before the end of the fall semester, with his approval, his attendance at the clinic was no longer required except when desired. Marvin acknowledged that his good speech progress related directly to his use of the opportunities that provided meaningful speech gratification experiences in situations consistent with his interests and and vocational aspirations. Marvin was overtly motivated to continue his progress. He had high regard for the assistance he had received, as well as the confidence shown by others in him, including students who, 'Did not look upon me like I was some retarded freak, or something to be tolerated. Perhaps, they saw me as I came to look upon myself'.

Case C

Bennett was a 41-year-old man with a pleasant outgoing manner. He exhibited moderate stuttering behaviors, with minor associated facial movements. He is married and presently employed with an insurance company.

Bennett's wife had called the clinic to inquire about 'curing stuttering with the Edinburgh Masker'. She had been informed about this device by a friend, who had given her an article, which called attention to its advantages for use with stutterers. An appointment was recommended for both her and her husband to visit the clinic for a discussion and demonstration of the device. At his wife's urging, they visited our clinic.

At the time Bennett had attended public school, speech therapy programs were not as yet available in his school district. He was, however, at the age of 7 years, placed in a special education class for half a school year. He stated that his stuttering was worse during his earlier years, and he had been subjected to considerable taunting by older boys. He has an MBA degree in Business Administration, and a minor in Economics.

Bennett's first formal participation in a speech therapy program was during his freshman year within at the university's speech and hearing clinic. His major advisor referred him for speech therapy. He regarded the program as having provided little consistent fluency improvement, but that it did help to provide him with a better attitude and adjustment towards being a stutterer.

On graduation, he had problems, in spite of good grades, in obtaining suitable employment, which he regarded to be the result of his stuttering. He had applied for a position with several large organizations for the experience and opportunities for advancement. He had five jobs with smaller organizations before his present position. He regarded his work with these organizations as, 'I was just spinning my wheels at routine clerical tasks, which a monkey could do for a fraction in peanuts'.

Bennett had been at his present position with an insurance company for the last 12 years, preparing actuarial and budget assessments. Bennett liked working at the company, but contended that he might have been given more serious consideration for a managerial position if he did not stutter. Then, he could offer his family more advantages. He regarded using the telephone as one of his major problems.

Bennett had also attended a private clinic program some 10 years before visiting our clinic, which he said had produced no consistent beneficial therapy results. His more recent efforts were taken from the Speech Foundation's handbook, *Self-therapy for the Adult Stutterer* (Fraser, 1988). The earlier comment, likening the handbook's abundance to therapy methods 'to learning to swim in a shower', was made by Bennett.

On discussion of our program, which included the concepts of shared responsibilities and providing opportunities for meaningful speech gratifying experiences, and the availability, objectives and demonstration of the Edinburgh Masker, Bennett agreed to a trial period consisting of two sessions. He was pleasantly surprised on listening to recordings of his initial fluent speech experiences while using the device. He also expressed surprise that no manipulation or related techniques, common to his previous clinic experiences, were required. We discussed his complaints and feelings regarding efforts to apply these techniques, as well as self-administered coping adjustment methods of his own.

Bennett was pleased at how readily he adapted to the device to gain notable increase in his fluent speech. He found it very helpful in its use with the telephone and decided to purchase an Edinburgh Masker. With his approval, different students (from our classes on stuttering, and unknown to him at first) were assigned to telephone him during the early evening hours. With prudence, the students could decide on the topic to be discussed. Bennett reported that he very much welcomed and enjoyed the challenge of these calls.

By the end of the third week, he was wearing his own device daily, particularly at work, and within town. Bennett was very diligent in his use of the device. He took every opportunity to phone or visit various stores and local public offices. His experiences were discussed at length within the sessions, with regard to assessments of his anticipations, feelings, emotions and, particularly, the successes derived from his participation in these speech experiences.

Bennett had decided that he preferred to bring his participation in our program, and the use of the masker, to the attention of his employers himself, which he did after purchasing the device. He reported that they were pleased at the evident increase in his fluent speech and his efforts to improve himself. He was encouraged to expand his work duties to be a more effective and responsible employee. He stated that this meant assuming duties that required enhancement of his communication skills. He was quite pleased to have chosen to do this on his own.

By the end of the fourth week, he was requested not to use the device during clinic sessions. Although hesitant at first, when listening to recordings of these sessions he was pleased with the apparent consistency of his fluent speech. He referred to his growing speech gratification experiences, and more readily available fluent speech, without the need to be concerned about various confusing coping adjustment techniques for maintenance of these experiences. He stated that replaying the tapes of our sessions at home helped very much. One of the objectives of openly taping these sessions was to discourage his preoccupation with them while speaking or anticipating speech.

At the eighth week, to provide more realistic, as well as meaningful, success opportunities for speech gratification experiences, it was arranged for Bennett to lecture on various aspects of the insurance profession before two classes within the university's school of business. (The students were not informed of his stuttering.) It was necessary to obtain permission from his office manager. He chose to do this himself, and was obligingly granted this.

In spite of his initial nervousness, he reported being pleased with his efforts, as were the students and class professors. After his third and last lecture before his civic club two weeks later, Bennett commented, 'I never imagined I could enjoy speaking publically so much. At times, I forgot I was wearing the masker' which he used sparingly during the third lecture.

By the twelfth week, Bennett reported relatively consistent fluent speech experiences at work, with reduced use of the masker. His clinic sessions were reduced to once a week and, with his approval, terminated 3 weeks later. Follow-up reports verified consistent stabilization in his readiness SET for performing developed fluent speech within his social and work activities, without undue dependence on the device.

Comments: it is to be noted that neither our clinic program nor my private practice solicited or profited from clients' purchases of these devices. The primary relationship with the dealers was limited to assuring the reliability of our clinic's devices, and those purchased by the clients. The clients' confidence in the devices was necessary to dispel the negative influences of distracting preoccupations with their proper functions.

Halmrast Senter for Stammebehandling, Norway

Norway has, for over 40 years, provided remedial programs for its young and adult stutterers. One of its main centers, Halmrast Senter for Stammebehandling, was regarded as a most uniquely progressive residential school for treating young and adult male and female stutterers. It might well have been singular among the world programs for treating stuttering.

Halmrast Senter provided comprehensive therapy programs, supported by psychological, social services and educational training. In addition, these services were complemented by social and recreational activities: sports, parties and trips to various places of interest, including trips to other countries. Field trips to local communities also served to provide contact speech experiences. For the young students, its educational program assured uninterrupted continuation of their community school programs.

All services at Halmrast are provided without cost to its residents. This includes travel expenses, from anywhere in Norway, between the participants' homes and the center. To maintain family contacts, periodic holiday and summer home visitations were provided. Adult residents are permitted leave from their jobs to participate in these programs, without loss of income. Halmrast provides its residents with a certain sense of positive social awareness, particularly because they do not have to cope with their problems alone, and because it provides the opportunity to return when the need arises.

One of the progressive results of Halmrast's multiple programs was evident in its residents being less likely to show stigmatization and/or to be disadvantaged from opportunities to pursue their interests and aspirations, particularly at the higher educational and vocational levels. The center's training programs were designed to motivate and support the residents more stable psychosocial adjustments by endeavoring to meet individual personal–social needs, while also endeavoring to treat the stuttering behaviors.

The service and activity programs at the Halmrast Senter might not have met all the needs of its residents. Severe stutterers might have only limited gains in speech fluency, in spite of having attended several times. Nevertheless, it was quite apparent that they benefited in self-confidence and emotional stability. Halmrast's comprehensive programs have demonstrated what might be achieved when stutterers are accorded opportunities that provided them with a motivating sense of personal worth and an awareness of a shared public responsibility expended on their behalf.

Perhaps, comparable comprehensive programs might not be as feasible for other nations to imitate, because of varying circumstances of population, size, economics, etc. Norway, however, had clearly demonstrated the validity of shared responsibility in providing ample opportunities for speech gratification experiences and treating the problems of stutterers realistically and with dignity. It is deemed most unfortunate, therefore, that Norway has succumbed to the theoretical whims of glib reformers, whose reforms trade human needs and a very beneficial and workable program for pragmatic political expediency.

Summary and conclusions

Speech is an essential social tool upon which we are dependent throughout our lives. It is a most valued tool for obtaining gratification, which, like good health, is commonly taken for granted until disturbed.

Threats to its use and dependence can be manifested as a psychosocial behavioral disorder, such as stuttering, which may cause people to be disadvantaged and, thus, subject to serious deprivation of needs and desired objectives throughout their lives.

Stuttering is thus not a form of speech disorder and it cannot be treated as such. Stuttering behaviors relate rather to concepts of the neuropsychology of human behavior. It should therefore be treated as a psychosocial behavioral disorder evoked by traumatic neuropsychological reactions to disturbed perceptions and responses to negative external stimuli. These reactions become manifest as episodes of non-speech motor behaviors, disruptive to the individual's natural availability of his developed speech.

Public attitudes, although generally slow to change, tend to be influenced by its professional members. Clinic programs, therefore, by actively sharing in the responsibility for the results of their therapy approaches for treating stuttering, can provide an essential link to the public, and thus assist their clients receiving the necessary speech gratification experiences, within the context of opportunities consistent with their needs, talents and desired vocations.

Demosthenes had more going for him than pebbles and the masking sound of ocean waves. He had the motivating opportunities of education and public office, which provided opportunities to experience speech gratifications not from his self-therapy techniques, but from the successes derived from participating in these opportunities. It is doubtful that he was not well aware of these essential psychosocial advantages.

Knowledge of stuttering, whether presented within this book or in other books, becomes useless unless used to promote understanding. Understanding is best measured by the extent to which it can be directed to the benefit of stutterers, which, in turn, benefits the public.

It has often been stated that, without proper knowledge of the basic cause(s) of stuttering, provision of consistent beneficial therapy will remain difficult. Yet, today, thousands of public and private clinic programs are attempting to do something worth doing, i.e. provide beneficial therapy for stuttering, without definitive knowledge of its basic cause(s).

There are, however, current methods for treating stuttering that are not being done poorly, but rather, I suggest, incompletely. We do have sufficient knowledge of the negative basic psychosocial factors that contribute in large to the stutterers' repertoires of neurophysiological dysfluency behaviors, and the repeated episodes of these behaviors. A major problem does not therefore appear to be insufficient knowledge, but rather the lack of sufficient inclination towards proper application of what is known with the means available.

To continue to subject stutterers primarily to self-control/manipulative and related coping techniques is contrary to the basic concepts of the neuropsychology of human behaviors and tends to reflect a kind of negative compromise:

> If we cannot tame or remove this beast from within the stutterer, might we not teach him/her to learn to live with it?

However, has not the real problem always been, and still is:

> Can we learn to live with the stutterer, whom we have made to live too much alone with the beast?

To re-phrase the opening line of this book:

IT IS HOPED I HAVE BEEN HEARD AND, I TRUST, BELIEVED.

Appendix I: Gerhardt

Gerhardt asserted that neither genetic and congenital nor post-birth deficits could account mainly for the many reading and related perceptual–motor problems encountered. He held that perceptual–motor disturbances occur primarily as a consequence of disturbed sensory–perceptual experiences. Gerhardt related neurophysiological concepts to disturbed reading behaviors. Acknowledging the genetic specificity for basic reading skills, he agreed with the Lurias that the genetic potentials for developing reading skills could be greatly influenced by external stimuli. In this regard, he provided interesting insights into the potential of external stimuli to have a negative influence on the development of specific perceptual–motor skills, such as reading and speech:

> External influences could 'selectively' affect the formation of specific skills, rather than constitute a 'generalized disturbance to the formation of a variety of skills'.

Gerhardt maintained that the proper performance of basic skills, such as reading and speech, starts with perceptions that closely relate to the fluency of the movements that are particular to the performances of the skill. He defined each step as a link in the 'chain of production' for the specific skill as follows:

- Object(s) of perception: the object, person, symbol, response or other external stimuli, perceived by the sensory modalities: vision, hearing, tactile, etc.
- Modes of perception: the temporal sequencing (order of the directional laterality) of the movements of the sensory modalities in their perceptions of the object(s) of perception, and transmitted as sensory excitations to the specific neuronal centers where identity is perceived.
- Temporal sequencing of the perceptual–motor movements: this

determines the sequences, as well as spatial order, of the perceptual–motor movements of the muscle systems related to the performances of the intended skill.

The patterns of the neurophysiological movements of the skill, formed within the respective neural assemblies, serve as the internal reference for determining the temporal sequencing (i.e. the timing and order) of the muscle movements for the performances of the particular skill or behaviors. (This has been discussed further as motor programs in Chapter 4.)

Gerhardt's neurophysiological model advanced his conviction that children, with no prior known inherent, congenital or post-birth defects, could incur reading disorders. Such disorders, he held, would more logically relate to the disturbing effects of ambiguous perceptions of external stimuli on the basic neurophysiological perceptual–motor processes for reading.

In summary Gerhardt, through his neurophysiological (chain of production) model, endeavored to show that the neurophysiological perceptual–motor processes remained comparatively similar, whether the child developed normal or disturbed reading levels. His holistic approach to perceptual–motor dysfunctions served as a basis for the formation of stuttering behaviors in Chapter 4.

Appendix II: Additional definitions and etiologies for dyslexia

Critchley (1964) isolated a category of reading disturbance that he defined as 'developmentally genetically determined'. He labeled these specific developmental dyslexia. This category is regarded to comprise only a relatively small number of the total incidences of reading disturbances, and was defined by the World Federation on Neurology as specific developmental dyslexia:

> A disorder manifested by difficulty in learning to read despite conventional instruction, adequate intelligence, and social–cultural opportunities. It is independent from fundamental cognitive disabilities which are frequently of constitutional origin.

Boder (1971) clinically classified three dyslexic subgroups listed below which are apparently classified on the bases of functional symptoms, rather than according to assumed etiological factors.

Dysphonic–dyslexic group

Children in this group exhibit difficulties in sound–symbol integration and in developing phonic skills. These children seem unable to sound out, or to end, the elemental component letters or syllables of a word. They can read words better in context than separately, and to guess at words from minimal clues, selecting words closest in meaning, but phonetically different from words that they may be attempting to read.

Dyseidetic–dyslexic group

This includes children exhibiting laborious efforts at reading. They seem to be seeing each word for the first time, but have difficulty learning what that letter looks like. These children are regarded to have poor visual memory, and are prone to read by ear, using acoustic phonetic bases for sounding out familiar words and familiar letter combinations.

Mixed dysphonic–dyseidetic dyslexia

These children exhibit problems with phonics and visual memory. They constitute the most serious dyslexic disorders because they cannot read, write or spell either visually or acoustically.

Turner's syndrome for dyslexia

This is attributed to sex-linked differences in children's processing methods for visual–special tasks. This syndrome was thought to be the result of 'gonadal dysgenesis', having only 45 chromosomes, the missing chromosome being an X of the XX pair. These children show visuo-constructional deficits: loss of space form and disturbed sense of directionality, which can be related to reading and writing disorders (Rosenthal, 1977).

The following overview, according to Lerner (1985), relates not only to its assumed cause(s), but also to the general tendency to view dyslexia in the biased light of one's professional discipline:

1. Heredity (Rutherfurd, 1909).
2. Incomplete cerebral dominance (Orton, 1937).
3. Impaired eye dominance (Dearborn, 1937)
4. Emotional bases. (Robinson, 1947).
5. Toxic causes (Thurston, 1955).
6. Environmental factors, socioeconomic (Vernon, 1958).
7. Pregnancy and perinatal brain damage (Kawi and Pasamanick, 1959).
8. Minimal brain dysfunction (Bax and MacKeith, 1963).
9. Delayed cerebral maturation (Critchley, 1964).
10. Nutritional factors.
11. Focal brain lesions.

Millichap and Millichap, as late as 1986, listed possible causes as follows:

- Biochemical: thinning of myelination of the nerve fibers (Duane and Rawson, 1975).
- Overloaded memory, weakness in short memory (Miles, 1993).
- Defects in the mechanisms for perception.

Appendix III: Kara and Roman alphabets

Kana alphabet

1. Each phonetic symbol, whether consonant or vowel, is pronounced and spelled exactly the same regardless of their position within the word, or with other words
2. No phonetic symbols (letters) have comparable 'mirror images' with any other phonetic symbol
3. No phonetic–symbol ambiguities
4. No 'whole word' ambiguities
5. No unstable 'script–phonetic relationships'. Each sound is represented by a single easily identifiable 'letter–symbol'

Roman alphabet

Many phonetic symbols, consonants and vowels are often spelled and pronounced differently

Examples:
give – logic
cough – through
malign – malignant

Has several mirror images
b – d
p – q

Has several phonetic–symbol ambiguities:
q – g
c – e – o
h – b
m – w

Has 'whole word' ambiguities:
was – saw
tab – bat
pat – tap

Has many unstable 'script–phonetic relationships'. Similar sounds are often represented by different letter–symbols:

f – cough – phone
k – can – clique
s – conceive
z – measure
su – sue – sure
n – know – gnome
ai – ay, aye, ei, eigh, eye, i, igh, y, ye

Regarding the contrasts between the phonetic–symbol inconsistencies and ambiguities of the English Roman alphabet, Hynd and Cohen (1983) stated:

> Japanese script consists of two series of Kana script (Hiragana and Kata-Kana), each consisting of 48 letters. It also has many ideographs, that are called Kanji script.
>
> Instruction in school begins with the Kana script, which is similar to our phonetic system. Unlike English, however, the Japanese phonetic system is constant in usage.
>
> Consequently, once the child learns the sounds associated with each Kana script, or the idea represented by the Kanji script, reading becomes an automatic process unencumbered by ambiguities associated with reading English.

A major consequence of this high phoneme-to-phoneme irregularity, according to Bannatyne (1973), was that:

> Since reading is very much an 'auditory-vocal process', the Roman alphabet may make it difficult for children to learn to read because they fail to properly remember its 'phoneme-to-grapheme coding system.

Bannatyne attributed this consequence to children's underlying higher cortical dysfunctions, such as deficits in auditory sequencing, memory, discrimination and phoneme blending, resulting from the inability to cope with the external perceptual ambiguities of the Roman alphabet.

Bibliography

Aiken, L.R. (1979). *Psychological Testing and Assessment*, 3rd edn. Boston: Allyn and Bacon.

Ainsworth, S. (1945). Integrating theories of stuttering. *Journal of Speech Disorders*, **10**, 205–210.

Arnheim, D.D. and Sinclair, W.A. (1979). *The Clumsy Child (A Program of Motor Therapy)*. St Louis, MO: CV Mosby Co.

Bannatyne, A. (1973). *An Auditory–Vocal Process*. San Raphael, CA: Academic Press.

Bax, M.C.O. and Mackeith, R. (1963). Minimal cerebral dysfunction. *Little Club Clinics in Developmental Medicine*, **10.**

Bender, J.F. (1938). *The Personality Structure of Stuttering*. New York: Pitman Publishing Corp.

Berry, M.F. and Eisenson, J. (1956). *Speech Disorders*. New York: Appleton-Century-Crofts.

Bloodstein, O. (1975). *A Handbook on Stuttering*, revised edn. Chicago: The National Easter Seal Society for Crippled Children and Adults.

Bluemel, C.S. (1960). *The Riddle of Stuttering*. Danville, IL: The Interstate Printers and Publishers.

Boder, F. (1971). Developmental dyslexia – prevailing diagnostic concepts and new diagnostic approach through patterns of reading and spelling. In H. Myklebust (ed.), *Progress of Learning Disabilities*, vol. 2. New York: Grune & Stratton.

Boome, E.J. and Richardson, M.A. (1931). *The Nature and Treatment of Stuttering*. London: Methuen.

Brown, S.F. (ed.) (1938). A study of stuttering in relation to various speech sounds. *Quarterly Journal of Speech*, **24**, 390–397. Originally published 1927.

Brown, S.F. (1945). The loci of stuttering in the speech sequence. *Journal of Speech Disorders*, **10**, 182–192.

Brutten, G.J. (1969). Stuttering: reflections of the two-factor approach to behavior modification. In B.B. Gray and G. England (eds), *Stuttering and Conditioned Therapies*. Monterey, CA.

Brutten, G.J. and Shoemaker, D.J. (1967). *The Modification of Stuttering*. Englewood Cliffs, NJ: Prentice-Hall.

Bryngelson, B. (1952). Suggestions in the theory and treatment of dysphemia, and its symptom, stuttering. *The Speech Teacher*, **1**, 131–136.

Bryngelson, B., Chapman, M. and Hansen, O. (1975). *Know Yourself, A Workbook for Those Who Stutter*. Minneapolis: Burgess Publishing Co.

Buhler, C.M. (1968). *The Course of Human Life: A Study of Goals in the Human Perspective*. Boston: Baker & Taylor Books.

Bullen, A.K. (1945). A cross-cultural approach to the problem of stuttering. *Child Development*, **16**, 1–88.

Canter, G.J. (1981). Observations of neurogenic stuttering. In O. Bloodstein (ed.), *A Handbook on Stuttering*. Chicago: National Easter Seal Society.

Carnegie, D. (1964). *How to Win Friends and Influence People*. New York: Simon & Schuster.

Carroll, Lewis (1968). *Alice in Wonderland*. New York: Random House.

Chesterson, G.K. (1938). *The Colored Lands*. London: Sheed & Ward..

Chesterton, G.K. (1985). *Orthodoxy*. Chicago: Thomas More.

Chomsky, N. (1965). *Aspects of the Theory of Syntax*. Cambridge, MA: MIT Press.

Chusid, J.G. (1973). *Correlative Neuroanatomy and Functional Neurology*, 15th edn. Canada: Lange Medical Publications.

Cole, M. (1978). *The Selected Writings of A.R. Luria*. New York: M.E. Sharp.

Coleman, J.C. and Broen, W.E. Jr (1971). *Abnormal Psychology and Modern Life*. Illinois: Scott, Foresmand & Co.

Cooper, E.B. (1968). A therapy process for the adult stutterer. *Journal of Speech and Hearing Disorders*, **33**, 246–260.

Crickmay, M.C. (1966). *Speech Therapy and the Bobath Approach to Cerebral Palsy*. Illinois: Charles C. Thomas.

Critchley, M. (1964). *Developmental Dyslexia*. Springfield, IL: Charles C. Thomas.

Curlee, R.F. and Perkins, W. H. (1984). *Nature and Treatment of Stuttering: New Directions*. San Diego: College-Hill Press.

Davis, D.M. (1939). The relation of repetitions in the speech of young children to certain measures of language maturity and situational factors. I. *Journal of Speech Disorders*, **5**, 235–248.

Dearborn, W.F. (1937). Ocular and manual dominance in dyslexia. *Psychological Bulletin*, **28**, 704–715.

Dickson, S. (1969). An application of the Blacky test: a study of the psychosexual development of stutterers. In O. Bloodstein (ed.), *A Handbook on Stuttering*, pp. 175–176. Chicago: National Easter Seal Society.

Dinnan, J.A., McGuiness, E. and Perrin, L. (1970). Auditory feedback: stutterers versus nonstutterers. *Journal of Learning Disabilities*, **3**, 209–213.

Duane, D.D. and Rawson, M.B. (1976). Reading, perception, and language . A study of the perseverating tendency in stutterers. *Quarterly Journal of Speech*, **22**, 626–631.

Eisenson, J. (1973). *Adult Aphasia (Assessment and Treatment)*. New York: Apple-Century-Crofts.

Eisenson, J. and Ogilivie, M. (1957). *Speech Correction in the Schools*. New York: Macmillan.

Eisenson, J. and Pastel, E. (1936). The perseverating tendency in stutterers. *Quarterly Journal of Speech*, **22**, 626–631.

Elkind, D. (1967). *A Sympathetic Understanding of the Child*. Boston: Baker & Taylor Books.

Fast, I. (1985). *Event Theory: A Piaget–Freud Integration*. ???, NJ: Lawrence Erlbuam Associates.

Fenichel, O. (1945). *The Psychoanalytic Theory of Neurosis*, New York: W.W. Norton.

Fisher, M.S. (1932). Language patterns in pre-school children. *Journal of Experimental Education*, **1**, 70–85.

Fitts, P.M. (1964). Perceptual motor skill learning. In A.W. Melton (ed.), *Categories of Human Learning*. New York: Academic Press.

Fitts, P.M. (1973). Perceptual–motor skill learning. In B.B. Wolman (ed.), *Handbook of General Psychology*. Englewood Cliffs, NJ: Prentice-Hall.

Fitts, P.M. and Patterson, G.R. (1964). Information capacity of discrete motor responses. *Journal of Experimental Psychology*, **67**, 103–112.

Fitts, P.M. and Redford, B.K. (1966). Information capacity of discrete motor responses under different cognitive sets. *Journal of Experimental Psychology*, **71**, 475–82.

Fraser, J. and Ainsworth, S. (1988). *If Your Child Stutters: A Guide for Parents*, vol. 11. Memphis, TN: Speech Foundation of America.

Fraser, J. and Perkins, W.A. (1987). *Do you Stutter?: A Guide For Teens*, issue no. 21. Memphis, TN: Speech Foundation of America.

Fraser, M. (1988). *Self-therapy for the Adult Stutterer*, issue no. 12. Memphis, TN: Speech Foundation of America.

Freeman, E.J. and Ushijima, T. (1978). Laryngeal muscle activity during stuttering. *Journal of Speech and Hearing Research*, **21**, 538–562.

Froeschels, E. (1964). Speech structure and stuttering. *The Voice*, **8**, 20–21.

Gerhardt, R. (1977). *The Writing Test*. Forsvarets Psykologitjeneste, Oslo: Mil/Akershus.

Glauber, I.P. (1958). The psychoanalysis of stuttering. In J. Eisenson (ed.), *Stuttering: A Symposium*. New York: Harper & Row.

Goldstein, K. (1939). *The Organism*. New York: American Book Co.

Goldstein, K. (1942). *Aftereffects of Brain Injuries in War*. New York: Grune & Stratton.

Goldstein, K. (1948). *Language and Language Disturbances*. New York: Grune & Stratton.

Gray, B.B. and England, G. (1969). *Stuttering and the Conditioning Therapies*. Monterey, CA: Monterey Institute for Speech and Hearing.

Green, T. (1991). Certain generalized responses of stutterers to psychologic tests. Paper given at International Conference on Stuttering, Paris.

Greenstein, T. (ed.) (1976). *Vision and Learning Disability Conference on Vision and Learning Disabilities*. St Louis, MO: American Optometric Association.

Hafford, J. (1941). A comparative study of the salivary pH of the normal speaker and stutterer. *Journal of Speech Disorders*, **6**, 173–184.

Hahn, E.A. (1941). *Significant Theories and Therapies*. Stanford, CA: Stanford University Press.

Hardcastle, W. J. (1975). *Physiology of Speech Production*. London: Academic Press.

Head, H. (1926). *Aphasia and Kindred Disorders of Speech*. New York: Cambridge University Press. Reprinted by Hafner Publishing Co., 1963

Hebb, D.O. (1949). *Organization of Behavior*. New York: John Wiley.

Hebb, D.O. (1959). A neuropsychological theory. In S. Koch (ed.), *Psychology, a Study of a Science*, vol. 1. New York: McGraw-Hill.

Hendricks, A.D. (1929). Cited in Hahn (1941).

Hynd, G. and Cohen, M. (1983). *Dyslexia: Neuropsychological Theory, Research and Differentiation*. New York: Grune & Stratton.

Johnson, W. (1944). The Indians have no word for it: stuttering in children. *Quarterly Journal of Speech*, **30**.

Johnson, W. (1947). *Toward Understanding Stuttering*. Chicago: The National Society for Crippled Children and Adults.

Johnson, W. (1949). An open letter to the mother of a stuttering child. *Journal of Speech and Hearing Disorders*, **14**.

Johnson, W. et al.?? (1959). *The Onset of Stuttering*. Minneapolis: University of Minneapolis Press.

Kawi, A.A. and Pasamanick, B. (1959). Prenatal and paranatal in the development of reading disorders. *Monograph of the Society for Research in Child Development*, **24**(4).

Keele, S.W. (1968). Movement control in skilled motor performance. *Psychological Bulletin*, **70**, 387–403.

Kelly, F.A. (1932). Some common factors in reading and speech disabilities. *Psychology Monograph*, **43**, 175–201.

Kessen, A. (1963). Cited in Pew (1966).

Kidd, K.K. (1977). A genetic perspective on stuttering. *Journal of Fluency Disorders*, **2**, 259–269.

Kirk, S.A. and Lord, F.E. (1974). *Exceptional Children: Educational Resources and Perspectives*. Boston: Houghton Mifflin Co.

Kolb, B. and Whishaw, I.Q. (1980). *Fundamentals of Human Neuropsychology*. San Francisco: W.H. Freeman.

Kopp, H. (1946). Psychosomatic study of fifty stuttering children: II Ozeretsky tests. *American Journal of Orthopsychiatry*, **16**, 114–119.

Krumboltz, J.K. and Krumboltz, J.B. (1972). *Changing Children's Behavior*. Englewood Cliffs, NJ: Prentice-Hall.

Laczkowska,M. (1965). *Painting in Stuttering Children*. (*De Therapia vocis et loquelae*, vol. I). XIIIth Congress, International Society for Logopedics and Phoniatrics.

Lemert, E.M. (153). Some Indians who stutter. *Journal of Speech and Hearing Disorders*, **18**, 168–174.

Lerner, J.W. (1976). *Children with Learning Disabilities: Theories, Diagnosis, Teaching Strategies*, 2nd edn. Boston: Houghton Mifflin.

Lerner, J.W. (1985). *Learning Disabilities: Theories, Diagnosis, and Teaching Strategies*, 4th edn. Boston: Houghton- Mifflin.

Linsay, P.H. and Norman, D.A. (1977). *Human Information Processing : An Introduction to Psychology*. New York: Academic Press.

Love, R.J. and Webb, W.G. (1986). *Neurology for the Speech-Language Pathologist*. Boston: Butterworths.

Luchsinger, R. and Arnold, G.E. (1965). *Voice–Speech–Language: Clinical Communicology: Its Physiology and Pathology*. Belmont, CA: Wadsworth Publishing Co.

Luper, H.L. and Mulder, R. (1964). *Stuttering Therapy in Children*. Englewood Cliffs, NJ: Prentice-Hall.

Luria, A. (1966a). *Higher Cortical Functions in Man*. New York: Basic Books.

Luria, A. (1966b). *Human Brain and Psychological Processes*. New York: Harper & Row.

Luria, A. (1973). *The Working Brain*. New York: Basic Books.

Maccoby, E.E. (1980). *Social Development: Psychological Growth and the Parent–Child Relationship*. Atlanta: Harcourt Brace Jovanovich.

Makita, K. (1968). The rarity of reading disability in Japanese children. *Journal of Orthopsychiatry*, **38**, 599–614.

Mandell, S.L. (1983). *Computers and Data Processing Today*. New York: West Co.

Martin, R.R. (1962). Stuttering and perseveration in children. *Journal of Speech and Hearing Research*, **5**, 332–339.

Martin, R.R. and Siegal, G.M. (1966). The affects of simultaneously punishing stuttering and rewarding fluency. *Journal of Speech and Hearing Research*, **9**.

McDowell, E.D. (1928). *The Educational and Emotional Adjustments of Stuttering Children*. New York: Columbia University Teachers College.

Meichenbaum, D. (1979). *Cognitive–Behavior Modification*. New York: Plenum Press.

Miles, T.R. (1993). *Dyslexia: The Pattern of Difficulties*, 2nd edn. London: Whurr.

Millichap, J.G. and Millichap, N.M. (1986). *Dyslexia: As the Neurologist and Educator Read It*.

Milner, P. H. (1970). *Physiological Psychology*. London: Holt, Rinehart & Winston.

Moore, J.C. and Rigo, T. (1983). An awareness approach to the covert symptoms of stuttering. *Journal of Dysfluency Disorders*, **8**.

Moore, W.H. Jr and Haynes, W.O. (1980). Alpha hemispheric asymmetry and stuttering: some support for a segmentation dysfunction hypothesis. *Journal of Speech and Hearing Research*, **23**, 229–247.

Mosse, H.L. (1982). *The Complete Handbook of Children's Reading Disorders*, vol I.

Moyer, K.E. (1976). *The Psychology of Aggression*. New York: Harper & Row.

Naidoo, S. (1972). *Specific Dyslexia*. London: Pitman House.

Nelson, S.E., Hunter, N. and Walter, M. (1945). Stuttering in twin types. *Journal of Speech Disorders*, **10**, 335–343.

Nolte, J. (1981). *The Human Brain: An Introduction to its Functional Anatomy*. St Louis: C.V. Mosby.

Ochroch, R. (1981). *The Diagnosis and Treatment of Minimal Brain Dysfunction in Children: A Clinical Approach*. New York: Human Sciences.

Orton, S.T. (1937). *Reading, Writing and Speech Problems in Children*. New York: W.W. Norton.

Palmer, M.F. and Gillette, A.M. (1939). Respiratory cardiac arrhythmia in stuttering. *Journal of Speech Disorders*, **4**, 133–140.

Patterson, G.R. (1971). *Families: Applications of Social Learning to Family Life*. Champaign, IL: Research Press Co.

Pavlidis, G.T. and Fishen, D.F. (1986). *Dyslexia: Its Neuropsychology and Treatment*. New York: John Wiley & Sons.

Pavlov, I.P. (1962). *Conditioned Reflexes: An Investigation of the Physiological Activity of the Cerebral Cortex*. New York: John Wiley & Sons.

Perkins, W.H. (1977). *Speech Pathology: An Applied Behavioral Science*, 2nd edn. St Louis: C.V. Mosby.

Perkins, W.H. (1978). Learning from negative outcomes in stuttering therapy. *Journal of Fluency Disorders*, **8**

Peters, R.W. and Simonson, W.E. (1960). Generalization of stuttering behavior through associative learning. *Journal of Speech and Hearing Research*, **3**, 9–14.

Pew, R.W. (1966). Acquisition of a hierarchial control over the temporal organization of a skill. *Journal of Experimental Psychology*, **71**, 761–764.

Piaget, J. (1952). *The Origin of Intelligence in Children* (M. Cook. translator). New York: International Universities Press. Originally published 1936

Piaget, J. (1968). *On the Development of Memory and Identity*. Boston?, MA: Clark University Press.

Preus, A. (1972). Stuttering in Down's syndrome. *Scandinavian Journal of Educational Research*, **16,** 89–104.

Robinson, H.M. (1947). *Why Pupils Fail in Reading*. Chicago: University of Chicago Press.

Rogers, C.R. (1947). Some observations on the organization of personality. *American Psychologist*, **2**, 358–368.

Rose, S. (1973). *The Conscious Brain*. New York: Alfred A. Knopf.

Rosenberger, P. (1980). Dopaminergenic systems and speech fluency. *Journal of Fluency Disorders*, **5**, 255–267.

Rosenthal, J.H. (1977). *The Neuropsychopathology of Written Language*. Chicago: Nelson-Hall.

Rousey, C.L., Goetzinger, C.P. and Dirks, D. (1959). Sound localization ability of normal, stuttering, neurotic and hemiplegic subjects. *AMA Archives of General Psychiatry*, **1**, 640–645.

Rutherfurd, W.J. (1909). Cited in Naidoo (1972).

Ryan, B. (1979). Stuttering therapy in a framework of operational conditioning and programmed learning. In H.Gregory (ed.), *Controversies about Stuttering Therapy*. Baltimore: University Park Press.

Schindler, M.D. (1955). A study of educational adjustments of stuttering and non-stuttering children. In W. Johnson and R.R. Leutenegger (eds), *Stuttering in Children and Adults*. Minneapolis: University of Minneapolis Press.

Schlanger, M.D. and Gottsleben, R.H. (1957). Analysis of speech defects among institutional mentally retarded. *Journal of Speech and Hearing Disorders*, **22**, 98–103.

Schuell, J. (1946). Sex differences in relation to stuttering, Part 1. *Journal of Speech Disorders*, **11**, 277–298.

Seligman, M.E. (1975). *Helplessness: On Depression, Development and Death*. New York: W.H. Freeman.

Shames, G.H. and Rubin, H. (1986). *Stuttering; Then and Now*. Columbus, OH: Charles E. Merrill.

Shames, G.H. and Sherrick, C.E. (1963). A discussion of nonfluency and stuttering as operant behavior. *Journal of Speech and Hearing Disorders*, **28**, 3–18.

Sheehan, J.G. (1970). *Stuttering: Research and Therapy*. New York: Harper & Row.

Sheehan, J.G. (ed.) (1970). The role of therapy. In *Stuttering Research and Therapy*. New York: Harper & Row.

Shopwin, C.D. (1959). An experimental investigation of the passive-dependency component in adult male stutterers (abstract). *Speech Monograph*, **26**, 143.

Shrum, W.A. (1984). A study of speaking behaviors of stutterers and nonstutterers by means of multichannel electromyography. In R.F. Curlee and W.H. Perkins (eds), *Nature and Treatment of Stuttering*. San Diego: College-Hill Press.

Silverman, F.H. and Silverman, E.M. (1971). Stutter-like behavior in the manual communication of the deaf. *Perceptual Motor Skills*, **33**, 45–46.

Speech Foundation of America (1985). *Conditioning in Stuttering Therapy: Applications and Limitations*. Memphis, TN: Speech Foundation of America.

Speech Foundation of America (1985). *Stuttering Therapy, Prevention and Intervention with Children*. Memphis, TN: Speech Foundation of America.

Strang, R. (1959). Cited in Lerner (1976).

Strother, C.R. and Kreigman, L.S. (1944). Rhythmokinesis in stutters and non-stutterers. *Journal of Speech Disorders*, **9** 239–244.

Toffler, A. (1970). *Future Shock*. New York: Bantam.

Travis, L.E. (1934). Dissociation of the homologous muscle function in stuttering. *Archives of Neurological Psychiatry*, **31**, 127–133.

Travis, L.E. (ed.) (1957). *Handbook of Speech Pathology*. New York: Appleton-Century-Crofts.

Travis, L.E. and Fagan, L.B. (1928). Studies in stuttering: III. A study of certain reflexes during stuttering. *Archives of Neurological Psychiatry*, **19**, 1006–1013.

Travis, L.E. and Knott, J.R. (1937). Bilaterally recorded brain potentials from normal speakers and stutterers. *Journal of Speech Disorders*, **2**, 239–241.

Travis, L.E., Tuttle, W.W. and Cowan, D.W. (1936). A study of the heart rate during stuttering. *Journal of Speech Disorders*, **2**, 21–26.

Trumble, D. and Noble, M. (1966). Motor skills. In B.B. Wolman (ed.), *Handbook of General Psychology*, pp. 188–205. Englewood Cliffs, NJ: Prentice-Hall.

Van Riper, C. (1935). The quantitative measurement of laterality. *Journal of Experimental Psychology*, **18**, 372–382.

Van Riper, C. (1954). *Speech Correction*. Englewood Cliffs, NJ: Prentice-Hall.

Van Riper, C. (1973). *The Treatment of Stuttering*. Englewood Cliffs, NJ: Prentice-Hall.

Van Riper, C. and Emerick L. (1984). *Speech Correction: An Introduction to Speech Pathology and Audiology*, 7th edn. Englewood Cliffs, NJ: Prentice-Hall.

Vernon, M.D. (1958). *Backwardness in Reading*. Cambridge,: Cambridge University Press.

Vogel, V. (19??). Stuttering cured by hypnosis. *Scientific American*, **151**, 311–313.

Wadsworth, B.J. (1971). *Piaget's Theory of Cognitive Development*. New York: David McKay Co.

Webster's New World Dictionary of the American Language (1970). 2nd College edn, edited by G.B. Guralnick (Editor-in-Chief). New York: The World Publishing Co.

Weiss, D.A. (1964). *Cluttering*. Englewood Cliffs, NJ: Prentice-Hall.

West, R. (1958). An agnostic's speculations about stuttering. In J. Eisenson (ed.), *Stuttering: A Symposium*. New York: Harper & Row.

West, R., Kennedy, L. and Carr, A. (1937). *The Rehabilitation of Speech*. New York: Harper & Bros.

Williams, D.E. (1957). A point of view about stuttering. *Journal of Speech and Hearing Disorders*, **22**, 390–397.

Williams, D.E. (1982). Stuttering therapy: where are we going – and why? *Journal of Fluency Disorders*, **7**,159–170.

Wingate, M.E. (1962). Evaluation and stuttering. *Journal of Speech and Hearing Research*, **27**, 106–115, 244–257, 368–377.

Wingate, M.E. (1964a). Recovering from stuttering. *Journal of Speech and Hearing Disorders*, **29**, 312–321.

Wingate , M.E. (1964b). A standard definition of stuttering. *Journal of Speech and Hearing Disorders*, **29**, 484–489.

Wingate, M.E. (1981). Sounds and patterns in artificial fluency: spectrographic evidence. *Journal of Fluency Disorders*, **6**, 94–118.

Wirschner, G.J. (1950). Stuttering behavior and learning: preliminary theoretic formulation. *Journal of Speech and Hearing Disorders*, **15**, 324–335.

Wischner, G.J. (1952). Experimental approach to expectancy and anxiety in stuttering behavior. *Journal of Speech and Hearing Disorders*, **17**, 130–154.

Wolpe, J. (1973). *The Practice of Behavior Therapy*, 2nd edn. New York: Pergamon Press.

Index